Clinical Decision Support: Tools, Strategies, and Emerging Technologies

Editor

ANAND S. DIGHE

CLINICS IN LABORATORY MEDICINE

www.labmed.theclinics.com

Editor-in-Chief
MILENKO JOVAN TANASIJEVIC

June 2019 • Volume 39 • Number 2

ELSEVIER

1600 John F. Kennedy Boulevard • Suite 1800 • Philadelphia, Pennsylvania, 19103-2899

http://www.theclinics.com

CLINICS IN LABORATORY MEDICINE Volume 39, Number 2
June 2019 ISSN 0272-2712, ISBN-13: 978-0-323-68115-5

Editor: Stacy Eastman
Developmental Editor: Laura Fisher

Reprints. For copies of 100 or more, of articles in this publication, please contact the Commercial Reprints Department, Elsevier Inc., 360 Park Avenue South, New York, New York 10010-1710. Tel. 212-633-3874, Fax: 212-633-3820, E-mail: reprints@elsevier.com.

Clinics in Laboratory Medicine (ISSN 0272-2712) is published quarterly by Elsevier Inc., 360 Park Avenue South, New York, NY 10010-1710. Months of issue are March, June, September, and December. Business and Editorial offices: 1600 John F. Kennedy Blvd., Suite 1800, Philadelphia, PA 19103-2899. Periodicals postage paid at NewYork, NY and additional mailing offices. Subscription prices are $274.00 per year (US individuals), $541.00 per year (US institutions), $100.00 per year (US students), $349.00 per year (Canadian individuals), $657.00 per year (Canadian institutions), $185.00 per year (Canadian students), $404.00 per year (international individuals), $657.00 per year (international institutions), $185.00 (international students). Foreign air speed delivery is included in all Clinics subscription prices. All prices are subject to change without notice. POSTMASTER: Send address changes to *Clinics in Laboratory Medicine*, Elsevier Health Sciences Division, Subscription Customer Service, 3251 Riverport Lane, Maryland Heights, MO 63043. **Customer Service: 1-800-654-2452 (US). From outside of the US and Canada, call 1-314-447-8871. Fax: 1-314-447-8029. E-mail: journalscustomerservice-usa@elsevier.com (for print support) or journalsonlinesupport-usa@elsevier.com (for online support).**

Clinics in Laboratory Medicine is covered in *EMBASE/Exerpta Medica, MEDLINE/PubMed (Index Medicus), Cinahl, Current Contents/Clinical Medicine, BIOSIS and ISI/BIOMED.*

Contributors

EDITOR-IN-CHIEF

MILENKO JOVAN TANASIJEVIC, MD, MBA
Vice Chair for Clinical Pathology and Quality, Department of Pathology, Director of Clinical Laboratories, Brigham and Women's Hospital, Dana-Farber Cancer Institute, Associate Professor of Pathology, Harvard Medical School, Boston, Massachusetts, USA

EDITOR

ANAND S. DIGHE, MD, PhD
Associate Professor, Department of Pathology, Massachusetts General Hospital, Harvard Medical School, Boston, Massachusetts, USA

AUTHORS

ADA AITA, PhD
Department of Laboratory Medicine, University-Hospital of Padova, Department of Medicine - DIMED, University of Padova, Padova, Italy

JASON M. BARON, MD
Assistant Professor, Department of Pathology, Massachusetts General Hospital, Harvard Medical School, Boston, Massachusetts, USA

ANAND S. DIGHE, MD, PhD
Associate Professor, Department of Pathology, Massachusetts General Hospital, Harvard Medical School, Boston, Massachusetts, USA

BRIAN R. JACKSON, MD, MS
Associate Professor of Pathology (Clinical), University of Utah, Medical Director of Support Services, IT and Business Development, ARUP Laboratories, Salt Lake City, Utah, USA

NIKLAS KRUMM, MD, PhD
Resident, Department of Laboratory Medicine, University of Washington, Seattle, Washington, USA

DANIELLE E. KURANT, MD
Clinical Fellow, Department of Pathology, Massachusetts General Hospital, Harvard Medical School, Boston, Massachusetts, USA

BRUCE P. LEVY, MD
CPE, Associate Chief Medical Informatics Officer, Education and Research, Geisinger Health, Danville, Pennsylvania, USA; Professor, Geisinger Commonwealth School of Medicine, Scranton, Pennsylvania, USA

KENT LEWANDROWSKI, MD
Associate Chief of Pathology, Director of Pathology Laboratories and Molecular Medicines, Professor, Department of Pathology, Massachusetts General Hospital, Boston, Massachusetts, USA

ANDREA PADOAN, PhD
Department of Laboratory Medicine, University-Hospital of Padova, Department of Medicine - DIMED, University of Padova, Padova, Italy

MARIO PLEBANI, MD, FRCP
Department of Laboratory Medicine, University-Hospital of Padova, Department of Medicine - DIMED, University of Padova, Padova, Italy

GARY W. PROCOP, MD, MS
Director, Molecular Microbiology, Mycology, Parasitology and Virology Laboratories, Co-Chair, Enterprise Laboratory Stewardship Committee, Medical Operations, Professor, Department of Pathology, Cleveland Clinic Lerner College of Medicine, Cleveland Clinic, Cleveland, Ohio, USA

ANITA J. REDDY, MD
Co-Chair, Laboratory Stewardship Committee, Medical Operations, Respiratory Institute, Assistant Professor of Medicine, Cleveland Clinic Lerner College of Medicine, Cleveland Clinic, Cleveland, Ohio, USA

JOSEPH W. RUDOLF, MD
Assistant Professor, Department of Laboratory Medicine and Pathology, University of Minnesota Medical School, Minneapolis, Minnesota, USA

LAURA SCIACOVELLI, MSc
Department of Laboratory Medicine, University-Hospital of Padova, Padova, Italy

NEIL K. SHAH, MD
Clinical Associate Professor, Department of Pathology, Stanford University, Stanford, California, USA

BRIAN H. SHIRTS, MD, PhD
Associate Professor, Department of Laboratory Medicine, University of Washington, Seattle, Washington, USA

J. MARK TUTHILL, MD
Henry Ford Health System, Detroit, Michigan, USA

ALLISON L. WEATHERS, MD, FAAN
Associate Chief Medical Officer, Cleveland Clinic, Assistant Professor, Department of Medicine, Cleveland Clinic Lerner College of Medicine, Cleveland Clinic, Beachwood, Ohio, USA

Contents

Laboratory tests are an integral part of the electronic health record (EHR). Providing clinical decision support (CDS) for the ordering, collection, reporting, viewing, and interpretation of laboratory testing is a fundamental function of the EHR. The implementation of a sustainable, effective laboratory CDS program requires a commitment to standardization and harmonization of the laboratory dictionaries that are the foundation of laboratory-based CDS. In this review, the authors provide an overview of the tools available within the EHR to improve decision making throughout the entire laboratory testing process, from test order to clinical action.

Clinical decision support tools that involve improving test utilization should be jointly overseen by a laboratory stewardship committee and the hospital informatics team. The roles of these groups vary by institution and may overlap. This is a team effort and collaboration is a must. The effectiveness of these efforts in an institution depends on the receptiveness of leadership and providers, as well as the effectiveness of the associated committees. Examples of the challenges and successes of laboratory stewardship interventions that have been operationalized at the Cleveland Clinic that use clinical decision support tools, as well as associated literature, are reviewed.

In recent years, clinical decision support (CDS) systems have become recognized as increasingly important in assuring patient safety and supporting all phases of the clinical decision-making process. In Laboratory Medicine, CDS systems are usually used to drive test ordering and diagnostic prediction while combining IT components and staff skills. However, educational initiatives, user and provider feedback, and expert consultations should also be considered integral to CDS. The aim of this paper is to provide an overview of some important developments in CDS in supporting the clinical decision-making process and guaranteeing patient safety by reducing medical errors.

Overuse of clinical laboratory testing increases costs, contributes to iatrogenic anemia, and results in downstream costs, including unnecessary work-ups and treatments. Physicians order unnecessary laboratory tests because of lack of knowledge, the practice of defensive medicine and adherence to historical test ordering. Utilization management is increasingly important to control costs and ensure patients receive appropriate tests for diagnosis and management. Clinical decision support is essential for a successful utilization management program. Successful programs rely on clinical informatics to identify misutilization, implement interventions, and track effectiveness. We describe the role of clinical decision support in a laboratory utilization management program.

To achieve effective laboratory automation, analytical capabilities must be developed to support data analysis. This allows for effective development and deployment of decision support strategies within the automated laboratory. Practically, these take the form of dashboards, static and real time; workflow processes, such as autoverification; reflex protocols; and testing cascades, which reduce errors of omission and commission. This requires data from the LIS and middleware that enable sophisticated laboratory automation lines. This article addresses the historical, current, and future state of laboratory analytics using examples and offering a framework to organize thinking around analytical capabilities.

Clinical decision support (CDS) can greatly enhance patient blood management through optimizing ordering and providing patient-specific information. At present, modeling and prediction have small roles in inventory management; they will likely have increasing applications to help guide donor center collections based on real-time demand to meet more dispersed needs. Transfusion side-effects management for both donor and recipients is an area ripe for intervention by CDS to enable proactive actions. Last, CDS and broader prediction will 1 day function alongside and seamlessly along many of our major processes to create a human-computer symbiosis.

Genome-enabled or molecular clinical decision support (CDS) systems provide unique advantages for the clinical use of genomic data; however, their implementation is complicated by technical, biological, and systemic barriers. This article reviews the substantial technical progress that has been made in the past decade and finds that the underlying biological limitations of genomics as well as systemic barriers to adoption of molecular CDS have been comparatively underestimated. A hybrid consultative CDS system, which integrates a genomics consultant into an active CDS system, may provide an interim path forward.

Brian R. Jackson

Esoteric testing presents a broad range of opportunities to improve clinical decision making. To be effective, the knowledge support needs to be seamlessly embedded into clinical workflows. Reference laboratories are uniquely positioned to play an outsized role in laboratory decision support, in part because they are large repositories of esoteric testing knowledge and in part because of their resources and client relationships. To accomplish this, however, reference laboratories must develop strong capabilities to integrate content and logic into clinical software platforms, including but not limited to electronic health records.

Bruce P. Levy

Pathology has a large role to play in the proper development, implementation, and optimization of clinical decision support (CDS). CDS training must be supported by an educational foundation in clinical and pathology informatics. Educational opportunities are currently limited, but expanding, in the pathology residency space with Pathology Informatics Essentials for Residents. The use of an educational version of electronic clinical systems is an important educational tool to support the needed outcomes-driven and exercise-based informatics and CDS training. With the multidisciplinary nature of informatics, it is advantageous to include laboratory professionals in the training exercises as appropriate.

Jason M. Baron, Danielle E. Kurant, and Anand S. Dighe

Emerging applications of machine learning and artificial intelligence offer the opportunity to discover new clinical knowledge through secondary exploration of existing patient medical records. This new knowledge may in turn offer a foundation to build new types of clinical decision support (CDS) that provide patient-specific insights and guidance across a wide range of clinical questions and settings. This article will provide an overview of these emerging approaches to CDS, discussing both existing technologies as well as challenges that health systems and informaticists will need to address to allow these emerging approaches to reach their full potential.

CLINICS IN LABORATORY MEDICINE

FORTHCOMING ISSUES

September 2019
**Advances and Trends in Clinical
Microbiology: The Next 20 Years**
James E. Kirby, *Editor*

December 2019
Immunology Laboratory Testing
Vinay Subhash Mahajan, *Editor*

RECENT ISSUES

March 2019
**New Pipeline of Immunoregulatory
Molecules and Biomarkers in
Transplantation**
Indira Guleria, *Editor*

December 2018
HLA and Disease
Julio C. Delgado and Eszter Lázár-Molnár,
Editors

SERIES OF RELATED INTEREST

Surgical Pathology Clinics
Available at: https://www.surgpath.theclinics.com/

Preface

Enhancing the Value of the Laboratory with Clinical Decision Support

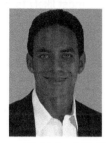

Anand S. Dighe, MD, PhD
Editor

It is 2019, and it is clear that the machines have won. Virtually all aspects of the health care experience have been, for better or worse, computerized. Within the laboratory, this has mostly been a positive development, with end-to-end barcode tracking of samples, advanced LIS systems, improved middleware, and analytics all improving patient safety and efficiency and enabling complex workflows, monitoring, and reporting.

On the broader electronic health record (EHR) front, many of the new laboratory-related workflows are still a work in progress. The ever-growing complexity of the modern EHR has facilitated both the need for clinical decision support (CDS) and the growth of CDS. CDS encompasses a variety of tools both within and outside the EHR to enhance decision making during the clinical workflow. CDS has the promise to improve the quality of care, reduce errors, enhance efficiency, and improve utilization and value. In this issue of *Clinics in Laboratory Medicine*, leaders in the field of CDS have written reviews that demonstrate the need, utility, and promise of CDS in virtually all aspects of the clinical laboratory.

The need for the laboratory to contribute to the EHR has never been greater. The rapid growth of diagnostic laboratory testing, combined with the ever-expanding amount of clinical data, has created a gap between practice and potential. Virtually all test-ordering processes are now within the EHR, and the EHR is often the only location where providers review results. The challenge for the laboratory is how to insert itself into these new workflows that are already shaping its future. One first step for "a seat at the table" is for the laboratory to fully understand the workings of the EHR. With this understanding inevitably comes the realization that there are in fact many opportunities for the laboratory to contribute to CDS.

Clin Lab Med 39 (2019) ix–x
https://doi.org/10.1016/j.cll.2019.02.001
0272-2712/19/© 2019 Published by Elsevier Inc.

To be accepted into the clinical workflow, CDS must deliver the right information, at the right point in the workflow, to the right person, and with the right format to optimize an individual provider's and patient's outcome. The modern EHR contains an array of CDS tools that impact laboratory workflows, including order sets, duplicate checking, search engines, passive information displays, result-reporting displays, alerts, templates, worklists, and reports. CDS is probably most associated with the dreaded interruptive or "pop-up" alert in the EHR. However, it is important to appreciate that often the best CDS is invisible and presents itself as a user-centered design of ordering and resulting workflows. Moreover, even the much maligned interruptive alert can be well received if targeted to the situations where the alert is most likely to be clinically useful.

It is important to remember that laboratory CDS is a team sport. The governance of EHR CDS often falls outside the laboratory, so it is essential that the laboratory demonstrates its value and works closely with the CDS team. CDS must be developed using a collaborative approach with analysts, providers, pathologists, laboratory staff, and project managers all playing important roles. A successful CDS program also requires a long-term commitment to continually evaluate existing CDS to optimize its value, as well as the monitoring of laboratory trends to identify new areas where CDS may be valuable.

Finally, it has been a pleasure to serve as guest editor for this issue of *Clinics in Laboratory Medicine*. I am extremely grateful to each of the authors for contributing their time, effort, and expertise to this work. I hope that this issue will give the reader a sense of how organizations are using CDS now to transform their operations as well as a glimpse into the future of CDS.

Anand S. Dighe, MD, PhD
Harvard Medical School
Department of Pathology
Massachusetts General Hospital
55 Fruit Street
Bigelow 510
Boston, MA 02114-2696, USA

E-mail address:
asdighe@mgh.harvard.edu

Decision Support Tools within the Electronic Health Record

Joseph W. Rudolf, MD[a], Anand S. Dighe, MD, PhD[b],*

KEYWORDS

- Clinical decision support (CDS) • Electronic health record (EHR)
- Computerized provider order entry (CPOE) • Decision support alerts
- Order sets/order panels

KEY POINTS

- Standardization and harmonization of laboratory dictionaries are a foundational step in creating a sustainable laboratory clinical decision support (CDS) program.
- Decision support for laboratory testing is not limited to traditional alerts and pop-up screens but encompasses all aspects of the laboratory testing process, including specimen collection and result viewing.
- Laboratory CDS requires a team approach with requisite knowledge of both the electronic health record and the laboratory information system as well as the infrastructure for building, testing, and monitoring CDS.

INTRODUCTION

The electronic health record (EHR) provides numerous opportunities for clinical decision support (CDS) for laboratory testing (**Fig. 1**). The ability to deliver effective decision support necessitates not only attention to EHR configuration and alert creation but also an infrastructure that supports monitoring, testing, and knowledge discovery. Herein, the authors discuss each of the laboratory-related elements of the EHR build that require attention to ensure that clinicians are optimally supported to make clinical decisions related to laboratory testing.

Disclosure: The authors have nothing to disclose.
[a] Department of Laboratory Medicine and Pathology, University of Minnesota Medical School, 420 Delaware Street Southeast, MMC 609 Mayo, Minneapolis, MN 55455, USA; [b] Department of Pathology, Massachusetts General Hospital, Harvard Medical School, 55 Fruit Street, Boston, MA 02114-2696, USA
* Corresponding author.
E-mail address: asdighe@mgh.harvard.edu

Clin Lab Med 39 (2019) 197–213
https://doi.org/10.1016/j.cll.2019.01.001
0272-2712/19/© 2019 Elsevier Inc. All rights reserved.

labmed.theclinics.com

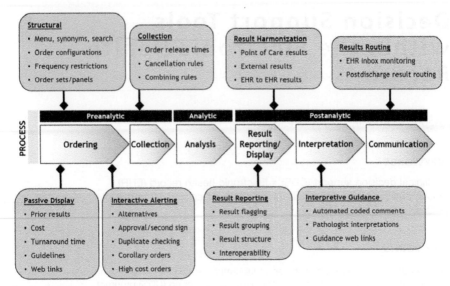

Fig. 1. EHR-based CDS in the laboratory testing process.

ORDER ENTRY
Computerized Provider Order Entry

Computerized provider order entry (CPOE) is a term given to the class of software applications that facilitate the electronic ordering of procedures, including diagnostic tests and medications.[1] CPOE began to replace paper-based order systems in the mid-2000s, starting with custom application development of "homegrown" EHR, and more recently, broad adoption of commercial systems. CPOE is a principal touch point for implementing CDS in provider workflows and confers several advantages over paper-based ordering. CPOE has been reported to be effective in improving laboratory test turnaround time, enhancing test utilization, reducing prescribing errors, decreasing redundant test orders, reducing patient length of stay, and, in certain settings, reducing mortality.[1–8] Although these reports detail positive impacts, achieving such success requires thoughtful design and implementation to be acceptable to end users. Poorly configured CPOE may increase provider cognitive burden, leading to fatigue and poor decision making.[9] Strong process governance and provider engagement are critical to successful implementation.[10,11] There are several passive and active tools for successfully delivering CDS in the context of CPOE, which are explored throughout this section. A summary of this section is presented in **Tables 1** and **2**.

Test Menu

When discussing CDS tools in the EHR, interruptive alerts (pop-ups) are likely the first tool that comes to mind. However, there are several other administrative controls that are both simple and highly effective. Of these, thoughtful test menu design may be the most important for the clinical laboratory. The decision of which tests to include on the test menu can significantly influence provider ordering patterns.[12] CPOE test menus can be finely tuned at a variety of levels, including the tests available to a particular facility and those available on department, specialty, or individual preference lists. They can also be managed through inclusion or exclusion from groupings of orders

Table 1
Electronic health record laboratory order entry considerations

Order Entry Item	
Item	**CDS Considerations**
Test menu	• Whether to include a test order as a structured EHR order on the laboratory formulary • Contexts in which to include the order (eg, facility, specialty, department preference lists) • Order inclusion on order sets and order panels • Miscellaneous order workflows for tests not on the structured EHR menu
Order configuration	• Restricting unwanted frequency configurations (eg, daily recurring orders) • Thoughtful default selections to encourage or discourage ordering • Preauthorization and second sign order workflows • Ask at order entry questions to facilitate timed draws (eg, therapeutic drug monitoring) • Configurations for add on testing
Search	• Standard test naming conventions for laboratory orders • Synonyms to increase search efficacy, including common misspellings • Including facility name if test is only available in certain locations
Passive information display	• Display of relative or absolute cost or charge data • Displaying test turnaround time • Displaying previous test results • Providing link to laboratory test directory (handbook) for additional test metadata
Interruptive alerts	• Configuring alerts as soft stops (available EHR override) or hard stops (no EHR override) • Discouraging duplicate orders • Suggesting alternative orders • Suggesting corollary orders • Presenting clinical calculators • Encoding guidelines

for care pathways (eg, admission or disease workup templates) in order sets or order panels. Well-designed order sets are effective in decreasing cognitive workload, promoting guideline adherence, streamlining care processes, improving efficiency, and enhancing user satisfaction.[9,13,14] A best practice for order sets is to limit the number of items on an order set because it is cognitively intensive for providers to assess large numbers of individual orders.[15]

Removing laboratory tests from contexts where they are not clinically valuable significantly decreases the use of those tests.[16–18] Because of the ever-expanding length and complexity of the laboratory test menu, in most centers it is not practical to have all available laboratory tests on the structured EHR order menu. It is thus important to have a robust miscellaneous test order process for requesting tests not offered through a structured order. The miscellaneous test order should include order entry questions to solicit specific information about the test to be performed, the collection container, and where the test is to be performed, all of which serve to reduce ambiguity upon specimen receipt in the laboratory.

Table 2
Checklist for electronic health record laboratory results display

Item	CDS Considerations
Result Display Item	
Abnormal result flagging	All abnormal result types (ie, numeric, text based) generate flags that are mapped to the appropriate flags in the EHR. Abnormal result flagging is present for all areas, including core laboratory, microbiology, anatomic pathologic condition, blood bank, and reference laboratory results
Delta result flagging	High-value delta checks (eg, increase in creatinine over baseline) are identified and generate flags or other strategies for alerting
Laboratory test result review groupings	The laboratory reviews the result groupings in the EHR for consistency and ease of review. New results are mapped into the results tree with laboratory input
Result structure	Result records are built with regards to related functionality, such as trending/graphing, reports, flow sheet display, and result population in clinical notes
Result status display	Key result statuses (eg, ordered, collected, received, in process, resulted) of an order are displayed in the EHR
POC results	Decisions are made regarding where to group, whether to trend with main laboratory tests, and how to label as originating from POC instrumentation. Manually entered POC results are clearly labeled as originating from manual entry
External results	Decisions are made regarding where to group, whether to trend, and how to label external results as originating from manual entry. All elements of a laboratory report are included in the externally entered results. Monitoring of external results is done to verify complete data entry
EHR to EHR results	Sufficient understanding of the outside laboratory's test methodology is available to inform decisions of trending and incorporation into CDS. A process for updates is mutually agreed on by the organizations sharing results
Result error queue monitoring	A robust process is in place that involves both the EHR team and the laboratory to quickly triage and address all identified errors
Result comments	Result comments are clearly displayed in all views of the EHR
Result communication	All ambulatory test results are sent to the electronic inbox of the responsible provider. Inbox monitoring is done to ensure result acknowledgment. There is a process for delivery and acknowledgment for results arising postdischarge from the emergency room or inpatient hospitalization

Order Configuration

Another passive tool for implementing CDS in the EHR is the configuration of individual orderable tests. Orders can be adjusted by users in numerous ways, including priority (routine or STAT), timing (now, with the morning draw, following the administration of a medication), and frequency (once or recurring). Default configurations are known contributors to ordering behavior, and preselected (prechecked) orders have been shown to be much more likely to be ordered.[19] If the desire is for an order to always occur in a given context, it should be preselected by default. It is important to make it easy for the provider to pursue the desired ordering practice. Selecting or unselecting defaults creates additional cognitive burden.[15] If a particular configuration is not desired, then that option should not be presented to the user. An example would be limiting the ability to place recurring (eg, daily) laboratory orders by removing the daily frequency option from the order configuration.[20,21]

Additional configurations need to be considered for specialized laboratory workflows. For tests requiring preauthorization or preapproval, it may be appropriate to include an entry order question soliciting the name of the approver. Alternatively, it may be useful to configure order routing to a pool of approvers, such as for high-cost genetic tests.[22] Limiting orders to a specified group of providers is another viable option.[23] In the case of second sign rules, for example, medical student orders requiring physician cosigning, automating this logic eases the burden on the cosigning provider. Orders may also be configured as batteries, groupings of individual tests as a single orderable item, or reflex protocols, where certain test results trigger additional tests to be performed, to further ease the ordering process.[24]

Timed draws and add-on tests may also require specific configuration. In the case of timed draws following a related event, such as the case of therapeutic drug monitoring following medication administration, CPOE order entry questions regarding the medication dose and time of administration are important data points to solicit. Add-on tests can be configured in a variety of ways with logic to permit the add-on only if a specimen is available and to trigger a new draw if no specimen is available in the laboratory. In the case of an integrated laboratory information system (LIS), it may be possible to alert the ordering provider to the availability of an existing specimen for an add-on to further enhance the decision-making process.

Facilitating Effective Search

Ad hoc orders, those not included in a care pathway such as an order set, require that the user searches for the item on the test menu. Search within CPOE is rudimentary when compared with commercially available search technology as implemented for the Internet. CPOE search typically relies on string matching, whereby the series of characters a user enters is matched directly to the series of characters in the order name or a designated synonym for the test. Misspellings or excess characters in a search may not yield the desired test in the search results. The process of search requires attention because if a user is unable to find a test with their search criteria, the test may not be ordered at all or an unintended test may be ordered.[25]

There are several EHR options that may be used to improve the utility of search. Standard naming conventions for tests can aid providers in their search.[26] For example, including "level" in the names of tests for therapeutic drug monitoring can help providers differentiate a laboratory test order from a medication order for the same drug.[27] Furthermore, adding synonyms for common misspellings, associated diseases, and alternative names have been shown to improve laboratory test search results.[25] Additional metadata included in the test name may also facilitate a successful search. If a given order is restricted to a specific site or provider group, it may be useful to include this in the test name.[27] Limiting the numbers of test variations may also be helpful to streamline ordering by reducing the complexity of search results.[27] EHR vendors have recently enhanced search technology within CPOE to allow for "fuzzy logic" matching when searching for orders and to enable searches that are able to simultaneously search for individual orders, order panels, and order sets in a single search. The authors anticipate additional emphasis will be placed on search in the future because search technologies common in other industries become increasingly adopted in health care.

Passive Information Display

The inclusion of passive data fields alongside the test name or within the body of an order can convey potentially useful information to guide ordering behavior. However, as the information is easily missed or disregarded, passive information about test appropriateness may not produce the desired changes in ordering behavior.[28] In one report, the display of the turnaround time for testing was effective at reducing send out test orders in the inpatient setting.[29] Displaying previous test results for a given order may also discourage repeat orders, although this has been studied only in the context of interruptive alerts, and not via passive display.[30] Display of test results relevant to a medication (eg, displaying the most recent potassium and creatinine when ordering furosemide) at the time of the medication order is also supported in many EHRs.

EHR ordering screens are typically limited in the amount of information that can be displayed. One means of providing more information regarding a given laboratory order is to provide a URL link within in the order to further information from a trusted source. Linking to an online laboratory handbook maintained by the laboratory may provide a convenient way to impart more information to clinicians.[31] An online laboratory handbook may include detailed information, such as test indications, interpretive advice, reference ranges, interferences, collection instructions, turnaround time, and cost.[31]

Inclusion of cost data and its effect on ordering behavior has been widely studied, and vendors have recently started supporting this functionality natively within their CPOE applications. To date, the results are mixed, with some studies showing no significant changes in utilization, and others demonstrating a modest reduction in laboratory test utilization.[21,32–37] When considering the display of cost to end users, it is important to assess which cost is the most appropriate cost to show. Options include the cost of performing the test to the organization, the potential cost to the patient in terms of the allowable Centers for Medicare and Medicaid Services charges, or the cost to a patient as determined by a separate fee schedule, such as the hospital charge master. Depending on the intended goal, the appropriate cost or charge to display may be different. It is also important to decide whether to display a relative cost (eg, $ vs $$$$$) or absolute cost (eg, $9.79). Some organizations may consider absolute charges to be proprietary information and disallow their display to end users. An organization may also have to decide whether to scale the costs of tests in a relative setting by area (eg, laboratory orders and imaging orders compared only with others in their procedure category) or whether there should be a single scale. In general, the authors recommend relative cost display scaled by area, because what constitutes an expensive imaging test is different than an expensive laboratory test.

Interruptive Alerts

Interruptive alerts are the mode of EHR CDS in which the workflow is halted to present information to an ordering provider, often through a pop-up window, and the user is prompted to complete an action before continuing. Interruptive alerts may be implemented as "soft stops," which allow the order to continue to be placed with an override, or "hard stops," which completely prevent the order from being placed. Both mechanisms have been well studied.

Soft stops have been successfully used to deter recurring laboratory orders, to recommend against nonpreferred or outmoded tests, to encourage corollary orders, to encourage awareness of expensive laboratory tests, and to discourage duplicate test orders within a specified interval.[38–54] These initiatives leveraged a variety of mechanisms, including indication solicitation, educational ordering information, encoding guidelines in the order workflow, displaying previous test results, cost display, and requirement of the use of clinical calculator.[38–54]

Fewer data are available on hard stops, but published studies have included initiatives to deter the ordering of multiple tests at a single time point instead of a stepwise manner, to limit genetic and genomic test orders, to reduce duplicate testing, and to limit hospital orders to certain frequencies.[23,30,51,55–57] Some hard-stop initiatives have included an option for provider override only by placing a call to the clinical laboratory.[30,57] Although hard stops have been shown to be more effective than soft stops,[51] hard stops tend to be less well accepted by providers.

Interruptive alerts should be used judiciously. As alerts increase in frequency, the likelihood of a provider accepting the recommended action decreases.[58] When a provider experiences alert overload, overrides may become subconscious and habitual.[59] The lack of specificity of alerts may contribute to alert fatigue and increased overrides.[59–61] The authors recommend limiting interruptive alerts whenever possible to improve adherence and provider satisfaction. When needed, tailoring interruptive alerts to very specific clinical situations and providers may be helpful in mitigating alert overload. Within a given EHR CDS build environment, there are typically numerous ways to customize alerts by using multiple criteria to restrict the alerts to situations whereby they are likely to be both well received and effective. For example, criteria, such as patient location, patient age, pregnancy status, provider specialty, diagnosis, medications, and prior results, may be used to target alert triggering to situations whereby it is most likely to be valuable. Another key concept in alert design is to trigger the alert as early in the decision-making process as possible, for example, triggering an alert suggesting an alternative laboratory order immediately upon selection of the triggering order, not at the time of signing, after the provider has spent time inputting other details regarding the order.

SPECIMEN COLLECTION

Numerous functions within the EHR play a role in the processes leading to specimen collection. For inpatient testing, there is typically a step in the EHR workflow where the laboratory order is "released" to the laboratory system to be available to generate specimen labels. The careful evaluation of the release times to be in concert with the collection workflows is necessary to avoid unnecessary, delayed, or missed collections. In outpatient areas, there is an analogous module in the EHR where previously ordered laboratory tests are "released" and specimen labels are printed. This step is a key area for CDS because tests may be ordered in duplicate, and in most cases, duplicate orders should be canceled. Moreover, the system should be designed such that laboratory orders that should not be collected until a future date (eg, a lipid panel that should not be collected until 6 months from the order date) or laboratory orders with specific instructions (eg, requires rapid transport to laboratory) should be highlighted to so that errors do not occur with their collection. Specimen labels should include specimen container information to reduce wrong tube errors.

The collection of "shared specimens" is problematic for many EHR and LIS systems. The issue typically manifests for specimens whereby several laboratories will be performing testing on the same specimen. For example, a pericardial fluid requiring testing for total protein, cell count, fluid culture, and cytology may be tested in 4 different laboratories (eg, chemistry, hematology, microbiology, and cytopathology), which may or may not share a common labeling or specimen collection system. Providing decision support for these specimens may involve using a common labeling system or standardizing the workflow for these specimens such that the first laboratory encountering the specimen has awareness of the need for the specimen in other testing areas.

RESULT DISPLAY

In the EHR, laboratory test results are typically displayed in grids or flow sheets to permit providers to more easily review related test results (eg, all the components of the basic metabolic panel are grouped in a specific location and displayed in a particular order) and observe and graph trends in test results over time. The "tree structure" or folders/subfolders of the results display grid provide important decision support to permit clinicians to quickly find and evaluate laboratory testing over time. For example, clustering all thyroid-related laboratory results (eg, free T4, T3, TSH) in a discrete "Thyroid" subfolder enables providers to see at a glance the relationships between the various thyroid studies over time. Although these folder structures are important to allow integration of test results, they create a potential patient safety issue if results that are supposed to be mapped to a given folder are mapped to the wrong folder or are not mapped at all and may fall to an "Others" folder in the result tree. These mismapped or unmapped results may be at increased risk of being missed by providers when reviewing laboratory results. A related issue can occur when multicomponent results (eg, lupus anticoagulant panel) are not reported together, creating a situation whereby the individual positive or negative components may be listed apart from one another, complicating interpretation. The use of EHR reports and tools to periodically monitor the system for unmapped or mismapped test results is recommended.

In the various EHR displays of laboratory testing, being able to visually highlight abnormal results is important to ensure that these results are recognized and appropriate action is taken. For quantitative results, flags on test results can be configured to describe the degree of abnormality (eg, a different icon for high, low, critical high, critical low, change from prior value). For qualitative results, such as microbiology testing, the flags are often set at the finding level, with certain organisms and findings generating abnormal or critical abnormal flagging. Some systems, particularly anatomic pathology or blood bank LIS, may have a limited ability to flag results as abnormal. Results generated from these systems (eg, Papanicolaou smears, antibody screens) thus may be at risk of being overlooked. In these instances, alternative approaches for applying flags to abnormal results may be needed, including using interface engine programming to evaluate test result values and applying flags to result messages before posting in the EHR. Another "blind spot" for flagged results may be results that are generated outside the primary LIS, including outside reference laboratories or directly interfaced results that bypass the LIS and are reported directly into the EHR. Interfaces from such laboratories may not send flags or may send them in a different format that needs mapping to the EHR. These interfaced results should be validated, and any deficiencies in flagging should be addressed.

Flags on test results, in addition to describing the degree of abnormality, can also be used to convey a significant change from a prior value (ie, a delta flag). The value of a delta flag for changes in serum creatinine has been shown to aid in the identification of acute kidney injury.[62] Moreover, studies that have incorporated the change in a test result value from its baseline or multiparameter analysis have also demonstrated value in alerting of a significant change in value that may not be flagged with traditional low- and high-value flagging.[63]

The ability to track and display the latest status of an order/result is an important mechanism to facilitate closed loop communication within the EHR. Without an updated order status being displayed in the EHR, providers will be unable to determine the disposition of the specimen, and duplicate orders and calls to the laboratory may increase. The EHR should be able to track and display the status of the key steps in the laboratory process, including specimen collection, in laboratory receipt, analysis within the laboratory, preliminary resulting, final resulting, and result acknowledgment.

Test results may be accompanied by comments to facilitate the correct interpretation of the test value. These interpretive comments may be automatically appended by the laboratory system based on the result value or may be created by laboratory staff or pathologists following review of the results. In several studies, both automatically applied and pathologist-authored comments have been shown to improve clinical care and laboratory operations.[24,64,65]

RESULT ENTRY

There are numerous results that are challenging to fully incorporate into the EHR. These results include point-of-care (POC) results, external paper reports, results transmitted from external EHR systems, and results converted from other EHRs. Unless these result types are entered in a structured, standardized format, they will be inaccessible to many provider workflows, and CDS tools within the EHR will not be able to use these results. The issues regarding each of these result categories are outlined in later discussion.

Point-of-Care Results

There are many challenges to including POC results in the EHR. The number and variety of instruments and their decentralized deployment complicate result incorporation into the EHR. Increasingly, POC instrumentation is capable of being electronically interfaced to the EHR, avoiding manual data entry processes that are tedious and may be prone to error.[66] Decisions that will impact CDS applications must be made about whether to trend POC results with analogous laboratory results or to present the POC results separately. These decisions are dependent on many factors, including the harmonization of the POC method with the central laboratory method and the reliability of the POC result entry process.

External Paper-Based Results

Results from laboratories outside the principal health care system are challenging to incorporate into the main EHR medical record. The source of these results is often paper laboratory reports, whether brought in by the patient or faxed or otherwise provided by another health care organization. If these reports are simply scanned into the EHR, the ability to provide decision support based on these results will not be present. CDS in all its forms, whether laboratory result trending, health maintenance, duplicate checking, or more sophisticated CDS, requires the external result to be entered into the EHR in a standardized, structured format. Even when standardized manual entry processes are used to enter external laboratory results into the EHR, it must be recognized that manually entered results are likely subject to much higher error rates than electronically interfaced laboratory results. As such, manually entered results should be clearly annotated as originating from manual entry. Furthermore, based on the confidence of the accuracy of the manual entry, consideration should be given as to whether to permit manually entered results to be included in the criteria that may trigger laboratory result-based alerting and related CDS.

External Electronic Health Record Interfaces

An emerging challenge is the handling of results from external EHRs that are capable of sharing data with the primary EHR. EHR vendors are increasingly enabling the sharing of laboratory data between institutions. With this functionality, EHRs can accept and file results natively to the EHR database. Although potentially of high value to an organization, this technology presents unique challenges, similar to trending Point of Care Testing, but at a much larger scope and scale. Given the differences between methods, assay cutoffs, critical values, and result interpretation between institutions, significant analysis needs to be done to decide which results to accept and whether to permit the data to trend with in-house assays. Standardized nomenclatures, such as LOINC, may be useful in mapping results between institutions. However, given the variation between organizational LOINC implementations, it remains to be seen whether this will be a practical means of automatically matching results. Although vendors may provide tools for mapping results between institutions, it is likely that a detailed comparison at the level of individual orders and results will be necessary. It will be important for the name and location of the reporting laboratory of the external order/result to be prominently displayed within the EHR to allow the provider to know the source of the laboratory data.

Result Conversion

During the process of EHR implementation or expansion, the conversion of laboratory data from one EHR format to another is often considered because it may be challenging for providers to use a new EHR system that lacks the historical record of the patient's laboratory test results. If it is decided that laboratory data conversion is needed, the conversion should be managed carefully because the laboratory result data will only be useful if they can be easily found and trended with existing data. Differences in the metadata describing the same laboratory test (eg, order name, result name, LOINC code) in 2 different EHRs can confound attempts to convert one EHR format to another.

COMMUNICATION

The EHR provides numerous opportunities for improving the communication of test results. The closed loop tracking of orders, from order signing to result acknowledgment, is an essential process for every health care organization. For laboratory testing, a key postanalytic step is the acknowledgment of the result by a responsible clinician. A common EHR approach for acknowledgment is to have test results routed to the EHR inbox of the provider that has been designated by the organization as responsible for test result follow-up. Within a provider's EHR inbox, it is important that results can be easily sorted and triaged according to criteria, such as result value flag, date/time, and result status. Test results that are generated postdischarge from the emergency room or hospital may need special result routing approaches to ensure timely acknowledgment.[67,68] Organizational monitoring of EHR inbox communications may be an important tool to ensure timely follow-up of test results.[69]

STANDARDIZATION

Many health care organizations consist of a network of federated sites. In cases where these organizations have grown by merger and acquisition, multiple clinical laboratories with different instruments and possibly different information systems (LIS and/or EHR) may exist. In these settings, the interoperability of laboratory orders and results is a significant concern and has profound implications for CDS. Harmonization is the process of standardizing methods, systems, reports, and result interpretation criteria.[70–72] This process is a challenging undertaking for institutions, requiring strong central governance and commitment. Accordingly, some enterprise environments have elected not to fully harmonize their clinical laboratories.

Nonharmonized systems face several CDS challenges. In the order entry process, providers may be confused about which test to order because test codes may not be shared among sites.[27] These orders may become inadvertently incorporated in orders sets/panels and individual preference lists.[27] CDS logic must be built and maintained to account for variation in codes and interpretation of results between sites. Result review becomes more complicated because results may or may not appear together within the patient chart and may not even be readily visible to providers at other sites. Lack of harmonization impacts nearly all phases of the testing process from order selection to result interpretation and increases the complexity of build maintenance within the EHR. When possible, the authors recommend harmonizing order and result codes, reference ranges, critical values, and reflex protocols between sites within an organization. As the prevalence and sophistication of CDS increases, the interoperability of laboratory data will become more necessary to support effective workflows.

INFRASTRUCTURE

The laboratory build is a central part of the EHR, with CDS, reports, note writing, and other key EHR functions dependent on the structure of laboratory orders and results in order to function properly. For example, providers wishing to automatically populate their progress notes with laboratory values will be dependent on the laboratory result structure that will identify tests to be pulled into the note. An essential element in the development of effective laboratory-based CDS is a laboratory team that is sufficiently familiar with the EHR environment to understand the various tools available to improve laboratory workflow and utilization. The laboratory team should receive training in the laboratory-related build of the EHR. Close working relationships between the LIS team and other key teams should be developed.

CDS programs for laboratory testing require environments where changes to the EHR and LIS can be tested. Ideally, the laboratory has access to several environments where changes to the EHR can be rigorously tested before moving the CDS build to production. The test environment should replicate the production environment as much as possible. For laboratory testing, the presence of active order and result interfaces between the LIS and EHR systems and the ability to create specimen labels are important to fully test laboratory functionality.

In addition to a robust test environment, the ability to work with test patients in the EHR production environment is highly desirable to provide a final check of new build.

The ability of the laboratory staff to view EHR ordering and resulting screens provides valuable insight into the need for CDS tools and the type of intervention needed. For example, laboratory staff can investigate why providers fail to order a given test by examining search results and the items included on order sets. In some EHR systems, a "shadow" copy of the production environment is available to selected users. This environment can be invaluable to debug challenging CDS objects because real patients can be used in a safe way that cannot impact the true production environment. The advantage of such an environment is that real patients may have the rich historical records that are required for testing complex CDS objects.

MONITORING
Order Use and Source

Monitoring the use of order sets and the CPOE origination location of orders (eg, order set name or preference list) provides a unique opportunity to improve CDS functionality. The authors have previously published a study outlining the development of a database including EHR order origination information.[73] This monitoring tool allows tailored interventions to improve order sets and preference lists when tests are incorrectly added to order sets (replacing red blood cell folate with serum folate), overused (replacing serum protein electrophoresis with immunofixation by serum protein electrophoresis with reflex to immunofixation), and permits the monitoring of orders for miscellaneous tests to determine when it is appropriate to build a structured order for a given test.[73] Monitoring the relative use of order sets may also be helpful for improving CDS. It has been documented that small numbers of order sets account for most of the order set usage. Understanding which order sets are most frequently used can help in prioritizing resources for optimization of the highest value order sets.[74,75]

Error Queues

Breakdowns in system-to-system interfaces may impact patient care and, because of the complexity of these interfaces, these errors may not be directly visible. For example, the failure of the specimen label for a single test to be printed due to an interface mapping issue may not be readily observed when a large number of other orders are being printed. System monitoring is required to identify and address these latent errors before they impact patients.[76,77]

Clinical Decision Support Alert Performance

Implementation of a CDS alert rarely signals the end of development. CDS alerts can malfunction a variety of ways, including correct design but incorrect EHR configuration, errors in CDS trigger criteria, and failures in rule maintenance due to newly added or discontinued procedures.[78] These malfunctions can lead to either false positive or false negative firing.[78] Although preimplementation monitoring of alerts, through so-called silent modes, where alerts are running in the EHR but are not displaying to end users, is useful, postimplementation monitoring is also a critical component of a CDS program.[79]

CDS monitoring reports capture data such as the rate of alert firing, the alert firing context, and provider characteristics of those receiving alerts. Regular review of monitoring reports provide a mechanism to proactively monitor alerts for sudden changes in alert behavior due to changes introduced during build updates as well as to identify opportunities to improve the specificity of alerts.[60,79] User reports are another common mechanism for discovering alert firing issues.[78] It is helpful to have a mechanism for EHR end users to share feedback about CDS firing so they can be investigated.[79] User feedback links can be included alongside the CDS message, decreasing the barrier to providing feedback. CDS dwell times (the amount of time spent with an alert open before selecting an action) may also be a useful tool for assessing CDS efficacy, although this has been less well studied.[80] Display and delivery of CDS monitoring data in a format that is both timely and intuitive for interpretation and action is a challenge. Increasingly there are dashboard tools both within the EHR and from external vendors that can assist in the visualization of data for assessing CDS performance.

SUMMARY

In this article, the authors have reviewed the breadth of CDS tools available in the EHR, including both passive and active tools for guiding provider workflows from order entry to result interpretation. They also addressed the underlying harmonization and infrastructure required to scale and stabilize CDS across an enterprise health care environment. When thoughtfully designed, implemented, and monitored, these tools can streamline care and decrease the risks of errors in ordering, processing, and interpreting tests. As the complexity of care grows and providers must attend to increasing numbers of stimuli, widespread CDS is quickly becoming an indispensable function to facilitate care delivery. Laboratory engagement and expertise are crucial factors in the operation of a successful CDS program, and the authors encourage all laboratorians to leverage the CDS toolkit for safe and effective care.

REFERENCES

1. Baron JM, Dighe AS. Computerized provider order entry in the clinical laboratory. J Pathol Inform 2011;2:35.
2. Georgiou A, Lang S, Rosenfeld D, et al. The use of computerized provider order entry to improve the effectiveness and efficiency of coagulation testing. Arch Pathol Lab Med 2011;135(4):495–8.
3. Westbrook JI, Georgiou A, Lam M. Does computerised provider order entry reduce test turnaround times? A before-and-after study at four hospitals. Stud Health Technol Inform 2009;150:527–31.
4. Schreiber R, Shaha SH. Computerised provider order entry adoption rates favourably impact length of stay. J Innov Health Inform 2016;23(1):166.
5. Schreiber R, Peters K, Shaha SH. Computerized provider order entry reduces length of stay in a community hospital. Appl Clin Inform 2014;5(3):685–98.
6. Prgomet M, Li L, Niazkhani Z, et al. Impact of commercial computerized provider order entry (CPOE) and clinical decision support systems (CDSSs) on medication errors, length of stay, and mortality in intensive care units: a systematic review and meta-analysis. J Am Med Inform Assoc 2017;24(2):413–22.
7. Rubinstein M, Hirsch R, Bandyopadhyay K, et al. Effectiveness of practices to support appropriate laboratory test utilization: a laboratory medicine best practices systematic review and meta-analysis. Am J Clin Pathol 2018;149(3): 197–221.
8. Bindraban RS, Ten Berg MJ, Naaktgeboren CA, et al. Reducing test utilization in hospital settings: a narrative review. Ann Lab Med 2018;38(5):402–12.
9. Zhang Y, Padman R, Levin JE. Reducing provider cognitive workload in CPOE use: optimizing order sets. Stud Health Technol Inform 2013;192:734–8.
10. Wolf M, Miller S, DeJong D, et al. The process of development of a prioritization tool for a clinical decision support build within a computerized provider order entry system: experiences from St Luke's Health System. Health Informatics J 2016; 22(3):579–93.
11. Fear F. Governance first, technology second to effective CPOE deployment: rapid development of order sets provides the foundation for CPOE, but healthcare organizations first need an effective governance plan built around clinician workflow. Health Manag Technol 2011;32(8):6–7.
12. Kim JY, Dzik WH, Dighe AS, et al. Utilization management in a large urban academic medical center: a 10-year experience. Am J Clin Pathol 2011;135(1): 108–18.

13. Chan AJ, Chan J, Cafazzo JA, et al. Order sets in health care: a systematic review of their effects. Int J Technol Assess Health Care 2012;28(3):235–40.
14. Avansino J, Leu MG. Effects of CPOE on provider cognitive workload: a randomized crossover trial. Pediatrics 2012;130(3):e547–52.
15. Zhang Y, Levin JE, Padman R. Data-driven order set generation and evaluation in the pediatric environment. AMIA Annu Symp Proc 2012;2012:1469–78.
16. Choi J, Atlin CR. Path of least resistance: how computerised provider order entry can lead to (and reduce) wasteful practices. BMJ Open Qual 2018;7(2):e000345.
17. Martins CM, da Costa Teixeira AS, de Azevedo LF, et al. The effect of a test ordering software intervention on the prescription of unnecessary laboratory tests - a randomized controlled trial. BMC Med Inform Decis Mak 2017;17(1):20.
18. Seppanen K, Kauppila T, Pitkälä K, et al. Altering a computerized laboratory test order form rationalizes ordering of laboratory tests in primary care physicians. Int J Med Inform 2016;86:49–53.
19. Olson J, Hollenbeak C, Donaldson K, et al. Default settings of computerized physician order entry system order sets drive ordering habits. J Pathol Inform 2015;6:16.
20. Iturrate E, Jubelt L, Volpicelli F, et al. Optimize your electronic medical record to increase value: reducing laboratory overutilization. Am J Med 2016;129(2):215–20.
21. Sadowski BW, Lane AB, Wood SM, et al. High-value, cost-conscious care: iterative systems-based interventions to reduce unnecessary laboratory testing. Am J Med 2017;130(9):1112.e1-7.
22. Dickerson JA, Cole B, Conta JH, et al. Improving the value of costly genetic reference laboratory testing with active utilization management. Arch Pathol Lab Med 2014;138(1):110–3.
23. Riley JD, Procop GW, Kottke-Marchant K, et al. Improving molecular genetic test utilization through order restriction, test review, and guidance. J Mol Diagn 2015;17(3):225–9.
24. Van Cott EM. Laboratory test interpretations and algorithms in utilization management. Clin Chim Acta 2014;427:188–92.
25. Grisson R, Kim JY, Brodsky V, et al. A novel class of laboratory middleware. Promoting information flow and improving computerized provider order entry. Am J Clin Pathol 2010;133(6):860–9.
26. Passiment E, Meisel JL, Fontanesi J, et al. Decoding laboratory test names: a major challenge to appropriate patient care. J Gen Intern Med 2013;28(3):453–8.
27. Petrides AK, Tanasijevic MJ, Goonan EM, et al. Top ten challenges when interfacing a laboratory information system to an electronic health record: experience at a large academic medical center. Int J Med Inform 2017;106:9–16.
28. Eaton KP, Chida N, Apfel A, et al. Impact of nonintrusive clinical decision support systems on laboratory test utilization in a large academic centre. J Eval Clin Pract 2018;24(3):474–9.
29. Fang DZ, Sran G, Gessner D, et al. Cost and turn-around time display decreases inpatient ordering of reference laboratory tests: a time series. BMJ Qual Saf 2014;23(12):994–1000.
30. Procop GW, Yerian LM, Wyllie R, et al. Duplicate laboratory test reduction using a clinical decision support tool. Am J Clin Pathol 2014;141(5):718–23.
31. Blechner M, Kish J, Chadaga V, et al. Analysis of search in an online clinical laboratory manual. Am J Clin Pathol 2006;126(2):208–14.
32. Schmidt RL, Colbert-Getz JM, Milne CK, et al. Impact of laboratory charge display within the electronic health record across an entire academic medical

center: results of a randomized controlled trial. Am J Clin Pathol 2017;148(6): 513–22.

33. Sedrak MS, Myers JS, Small DS, et al. Effect of a price transparency intervention in the electronic health record on clinician ordering of inpatient laboratory tests: the PRICE randomized clinical trial. JAMA Intern Med 2017;177(7):939–45.

34. Silvestri MT, Xu X, Long T, et al. Impact of cost display on ordering patterns for hospital laboratory and imaging services. J Gen Intern Med 2018;33(8):1268–75.

35. Ekblom K, Petersson A. Introduction of cost display reduces laboratory test utilization. Am J Manag Care 2018;24(5):e164–9.

36. Goetz C, Rotman SR, Hartoularos G, et al. The effect of charge display on cost of care and physician practice behaviors: a systematic review. J Gen Intern Med 2015;30(6):835–42.

37. Feldman LS, Shihab HM, Thiemann D, et al. Impact of providing fee data on laboratory test ordering: a controlled clinical trial. JAMA Intern Med 2013;173(10): 903–8.

38. Rudolf JW, Dighe AS, Coley CM, et al. Analysis of daily laboratory orders at a large urban academic center: a multifaceted approach to changing test ordering patterns. Am J Clin Pathol 2017;148(2):128–35.

39. Jackups R Jr, Szymanski JJ, Persaud SP. Clinical decision support for hematology laboratory test utilization. Int J Lab Hematol 2017;39(Suppl 1):128–35.

40. Ducatman AM, Tacker DH, Ducatman BS, et al. Quality improvement intervention for reduction of redundant testing. Acad Pathol 2017;4. 2374289517707506.

41. Chadwick DR, Hall C, Rae C, et al. A feasibility study for a clinical decision support system prompting HIV testing. HIV Med 2017;18(6):435–9.

42. Moyer AM, Saenger AK, Willrich M, et al. Implementation of clinical decision support rules to reduce repeat measurement of serum ionized calcium, serum magnesium, and N-Terminal Pro-B-type natriuretic peptide in intensive care unit inpatients. Clin Chem 2016;62(6):824–30.

43. Gottheil S, Khemani E, Copley K, et al. Reducing inappropriate ESR testing with computerized clinical decision support. BMJ Qual Improv Rep 2016;5(1).

44. Love SA, McKinney ZJ, Sandoval Y, et al. Electronic medical record-based performance improvement project to document and reduce excessive cardiac troponin testing. Clin Chem 2015;61(3):498–504.

45. Samuelson BT, Glynn E, Holmes M, et al. Use of a computer-based provider order entry (CPOE) intervention to optimize laboratory testing in patients with suspected heparin-induced thrombocytopenia. Thromb Res 2015;136(5):928–31.

46. McWilliams B, Triulzi DJ, Waters JH, et al. Trends in RBC ordering and use after implementing adaptive alerts in the electronic computerized physician order entry system. Am J Clin Pathol 2014;141(4):534–41.

47. Howell LP, MacDonald S, Jones J, et al. Can automated alerts within computerized physician order entry improve compliance with laboratory practice guidelines for ordering Pap tests? J Pathol Inform 2014;5(1):37.

48. Collins RA, Triulzi DJ, Waters JH, et al. Evaluation of real-time clinical decision support systems for platelet and cryoprecipitate orders. Am J Clin Pathol 2014; 141(1):78–84.

49. Levick DL, Stern G, Meyerhoefer CD, et al. Reducing unnecessary testing in a CPOE system through implementation of a targeted CDS intervention. BMC Med Inform Decis Mak 2013;13:43.

50. Baron JM, Lewandrowski KB, Kamis IK, et al. A novel strategy for evaluating the effects of an electronic test ordering alert message: optimizing cardiac marker use. J Pathol Inform 2012;3:3.

51. Procop GW, Keating C, Stagno P, et al. Reducing duplicate testing: a comparison of two clinical decision support tools. Am J Clin Pathol 2015;143(5):623–6.
52. Dunbar NM, Szczepiorkowski ZM. Hardwiring patient blood management: harnessing information technology to optimize transfusion practice. Curr Opin Hematol 2014;21(6):515–20.
53. Overhage JM, Tierney WM, Zhou XH, et al. A randomized trial of "corollary orders" to prevent errors of omission. J Am Med Inform Assoc 1997;4(5):364–75.
54. Riley JD, Stanley G, Wyllie R, et al. The impact of an electronic expensive test notification. Am J Clin Pathol 2018;149(6):530–5.
55. Dalal S, Bhesania S, Silber S, et al. Use of electronic clinical decision support and hard stops to decrease unnecessary thyroid function testing. BMJ Qual Improv Rep 2017;6(1) [pii:u223041.w8346].
56. Algaze CA, Wood M, Pageler NM, et al. Use of a checklist and clinical decision support tool reduces laboratory use and improves cost. Pediatrics 2016;137(1). https://doi.org/10.1542/peds.2014-3019.
57. Nikolic D, Richter SS, Asamoto K, et al. Implementation of a clinical decision support tool for stool cultures and parasitological studies in hospitalized patients. J Clin Microbiol 2017;55(12):3350–4.
58. Ancker JS, Edwards A, Nosal S, et al. Effects of workload, work complexity, and repeated alerts on alert fatigue in a clinical decision support system. BMC Med Inform Decis Mak 2017;17(1):36.
59. Baysari MT, Tariq A, Day RO, et al. Alert override as a habitual behavior - a new perspective on a persistent problem. J Am Med Inform Assoc 2017;24(2):409–12.
60. Lam JH, Ng O. Monitoring clinical decision support in the electronic health record. Am J Health Syst Pharm 2017;74(15):1130–3.
61. Carli D, Fahrni G, Bonnabry P, et al. Quality of decision support in computerized provider order entry: systematic literature review. JMIR Med Inform 2018;6(1):e3.
62. Garner AE, Lewington AJ, Barth JH. Detection of patients with acute kidney injury by the clinical laboratory using rises in serum creatinine: comparison of proposed definitions and a laboratory delta check. Ann Clin Biochem 2012;49(Pt 1):59–62.
63. Baron JM, Cheng XS, Bazari H, et al. Enhanced creatinine and estimated glomerular filtration rate reporting to facilitate detection of acute kidney injury. Am J Clin Pathol 2015;143(1):42–9.
64. Laposata ME, Laposata M, Van Cott EM, et al. Physician survey of a laboratory medicine interpretive service and evaluation of the influence of interpretations on laboratory test ordering. Arch Pathol Lab Med 2004;128(12):1424–7.
65. Schmidt RL, Panlener JJ, Carasso SM, et al. Impact of continuous improvement of laboratory test result comments on requests for consultation: a case series. Am J Clin Pathol 2016;145(5):666–70.
66. Nichols JH. Quality in point-of-care testing. Expert Rev Mol Diagn 2003;3(5):563–72.
67. Poon EG, Gandhi TK, Sequist TD, et al. "I wish I had seen this test result earlier!": dissatisfaction with test result management systems in primary care. Arch Intern Med 2004;164(20):2223–8.
68. Roy CL, Poon EG, Karson AS, et al. Patient safety concerns arising from test results that return after hospital discharge. Ann Intern Med 2005;143(2):121–8.
69. Roy CL, Rothschild JM, Dighe AS, et al. An initiative to improve the management of clinically significant test results in a large health care network. Jt Comm J Qual Patient Saf 2013;39(11):517–27.
70. Plebani M. Harmonization in laboratory medicine: requests, samples, measurements and reports. Crit Rev Clin Lab Sci 2016;53(3):184–96.

71. Plebani M, Panteghini M. Promoting clinical and laboratory interaction by harmonization. Clin Chim Acta 2014;432:15–21.
72. Miller WG, Tate JR, Barth JH, et al. Harmonization: the sample, the measurement, and the report. Ann Lab Med 2014;34(3):187–97.
73. Kurant DE, Baron JM, Strazimiri G, et al. Creation and use of an electronic health record reporting database to improve a laboratory test utilization program. Appl Clin Inform 2018;9(3):519–27.
74. Wright A, Feblowitz JC, Pang JE, et al. Use of order sets in inpatient computerized provider order entry systems: a comparative analysis of usage patterns at seven sites. Int J Med Inform 2012;81(11):733–45.
75. Wright A, Sittig DF, Carpenter JD, et al. Order sets in computerized physician order entry systems: an analysis of seven sites. AMIA Annu Symp Proc 2010;2010: 892–6.
76. Schreiber R, Sittig DF, Ash J, et al. Orders on file but no labs drawn: investigation of machine and human errors caused by an interface idiosyncrasy. J Am Med Inform Assoc 2017;24(5):958–63.
77. Sittig DF, Campbell E, Guappone K, et al. Recommendations for monitoring and evaluation of in-patient Computer-based Provider Order Entry Systems: results of a Delphi survey. AMIA Annu Symp Proc 2007;2007:671–5.
78. Wright A, Ai A, Ash J, et al. Clinical decision support alert malfunctions: analysis and empirically derived taxonomy. J Am Med Inform Assoc 2018;25(5):496–506.
79. Yoshida E, Fei S, Bavuso K, et al. The value of monitoring clinical decision support interventions. Appl Clin Inform 2018;9(1):163–73.
80. McDaniel RB, Burlison JD, Baker DK, et al. Alert dwell time: introduction of a measure to evaluate interruptive clinical decision support alerts. J Am Med Inform Assoc 2016;23(e1):e138–41.

Operational Aspects of a Clinical Decision Support Program

Gary W. Procop, MD, MS[a],*, Allison L. Weathers, MD, FAAN[b],
Anita J. Reddy, MD[c]

KEYWORDS

- Laboratory stewardship • Best practice focused • Decision support • Collaborative
- Non-intrusive • Functional • Measurable outcomes

KEY POINTS

- Leadership, organization, governance, and support are needed for success.
- Project management improves project completion and time to completion.
- Best practices in care delivery should be the driving force; cost-savings will naturally follow.
- Hard stop clinical decision support tools (CDSTs) are more effective than soft stop CDSTs, but a process to support provider overrides of an electronic blockage should be in place.
- Report generation and outcome measures demonstrate the effectiveness of interventions and are important to continue to foster support.

INTRODUCTION

A clinical decision support program does not usually exist as a stand-alone program. The request for the implementation of clinical decision support is often directed to the individuals overseeing the hospital and/or laboratory informatics services, but requests pertaining to laboratory testing may be directed to the staff of the laboratory. In many instances, these requests are from clinicians who are frustrated by the performance of the hospital or laboratory information system, respectively.[1] Alternatively, a conscientious provider, pathologist or laboratorian may notice over-, under-, or misutilized tests, and seek to use tools within the clinical information system to implement

Disclosure Statement: No disclosures or conflicts of interest.
[a] Molecular Microbiology, Mycology, Parasitology and Virology Laboratories, Enterprise Laboratory Stewardship Committee, Department of Medical Operations, Cleveland Clinic Lerner College of Medicine, Cleveland Clinic, 9500 Euclid Avenue/ LL2-131, Cleveland, OH 44195, USA; [b] Cleveland Clinic Lerner College of Medicine, Cleveland Clinic, 25900 Science Park Drive, AC220 Beechwood, OH 44122, USA; [c] Respiratory Institute, Cleveland Clinic Lerner College of Medicine, Cleveland Clinic, 9500 Euclid Avenue/ G6-156, Cleveland, OH 44195, USA
* Cleveland Clinic, 9500 Euclid Avenue/ LL2-131, Cleveland, OH 44195.
E-mail address: procopg@ccf.org

Clin Lab Med 39 (2019) 215–229
https://doi.org/10.1016/j.cll.2019.01.002
0272-2712/19/© 2019 Elsevier Inc. All rights reserved.
labmed.theclinics.com

some type of intervention. In such instances, the leadership of the informatics team, by default, assumes the governance responsibility for implementation and maintenance of these test utilization measures. The scenario described above is highly reliant on self-directed individuals, usually addresses a single problem rather than developing queue of process improvement initiatives, and may founder unless the individual desiring the change has patience, tenacity, sufficient experience, and/or authority to bring the project to a successful conclusion.

The scenario described above is reactive rather than proactive. One of the limitations with this approach is that agreement with the proposed intervention may not have been vetted with all medical staff, or with a group (eg, the laboratory stewardship committee) that has been charged to oversee such implementations. Another common challenge to this reactive approach is that the leadership of informatics, if not particularly dedicated to laboratory stewardship, may implement the requested intervention and then move on to the next task in their queue (eg, system upgrade, interface connections). Although the intervention was made, a determination of the efficacy of the intervention was not performed. This is one of the most significant shortcomings of this approach, because the lack of outcome measures deprives the academic community of evidence for or against such interventions and fails to inform hospital informatics and hospital operations regarding the return on the investment of such interventions, which do incur a cost.

In this article, we propose a collaborative effort between members of Pathology and Laboratory Medicine, clinical service representatives, hospital and laboratory informatics, and administration, as a means to optimize the use of clinical decision support tools (CDSTs) in laboratory stewardship. This approach has also been proposed by others.[2,3]

RECEPTIVENESS

Clinical decision support tools are often viewed as annoyances and, at worse, as impediments to clinical care delivery. The non-judicious use of CDSTs and poor governance of a clinical decision support program may justify such a characterization.[4] Ergo, it is critical that these tools are not implemented in a reactive or haphazard manner. Rather, these should be implemented after thorough consideration as to how these will affect clinical care delivery and how the use of such a tool will improve clinical care. As denoted above, it is the opinion of these authors that these decisions are best made in the context of a laboratory stewardship or similar oversight committee, which has appropriate representation from the laboratory, clinical services, and informatics.

Once a challenge has been identified for which a CDST is recommended, then the receptiveness of the individuals who will be affected by this intervention should be assessed, as well as that of hospital leadership.[2,3] It is best to review the proposal with hospital leadership to assure support before using resources to build and test the recommended intervention. If hospital leadership is not in agreement, then the leaders of the laboratory stewardship committee should meet with them to discuss the reasons for the intervention, the estimate of the impact on clinical services, and an estimate on the impact of the intervention (eg, decreased unnecessary phlebotomy).

If the hospital leadership is supportive of the intervention, then it is important to assess the receptiveness of individuals who will be affected by the intervention (eg, nurses). If the composition of the laboratory stewardship committee is broad, then there should be a sense of the receptiveness, because someone on the committee is from or associated with the affected area. If there is not someone from the area on the standing committee, then ad hoc members may be added for particular projects. This is an effective way to approach issues when expertise on the committee is lacking.[3]

If hospital leadership is not supportive, then perhaps additional data may be needed. A pilot project could be proposed or the project in question may have to be deferred or abandoned. It is important to recognize that all projects, even very sound projects, will not always be supported. It is important to not become discouraged by a lack of support. In such instances, it is important to reflect on the mission and recent important developments within the health system. Tailoring projects that align with the overall mission of the health system is a strategy to achieve support. For example, if a new cancer center is being constructed, then the use of CDSTs that assists oncologists in chemotherapy selection and prevent mistakes in dosing would likely be embraced.

GOVERNANCE

The PLUGS National Committee for Laboratory Stewardship has listed the key elements of governance as leadership commitment, accountability to a high-level medical executive, committees and subcommittees, laboratory experience, and other key support and networking.[2] Although there is not disagreement with these elements, the Clinical Laboratory Standards Institute's GP49 document, *Developing and Managing a Medical (Test) Utilization Management Program*, reminds us that one size does not fit all with respect to the size, management, and overseeing of test utilization initiatives, and that not having all elements in place should not deter utilization improvement efforts.[3] However, as committees grow beyond the size of one to a few individuals interested in, and performing, test utilization projects, then the governance of the group should become more formalized. This is also important for gaining legitimacy within the institution. The committee should have a Chair or Co-Chairs, who have enough experience and credibility at the institution to be able to promote the initiatives developed by the committee. The committee should also develop a reporting structure. These types of committees often report to Quality or Medical Operations, which go by various but similar names at different institutions. In many instances, there will be a dotted line reporting to Pathology and Laboratory Medicine, because this department is responsible for pathology and laboratory services within the health system.

The Chair may either be a pathologist or a clinician. A strong internal motivation and a dedication to optimizing laboratory utilization is more important than the particular training of the individual holding the position of Chair.

COLLABORATION WITH HOSPITAL INFORMATICS

Hospital information systems are effective vehicles for the implementation of a variety of interventions; a representative from the hospital informatics team should be part of the multidisciplinary laboratory stewardship team.[5,6] Although the focus of this work is on CDSTs, there are several methods or tools that may be used in conjunction with the hospital informatics team to improve laboratory stewardship. The applications, regardless of the complexity subsequently described, are usually maintained by the hospital information team. The CDSTs may come as a predesigned portion of the hospital information system, may be predesigned but require some customization, or may be a fully customized intervention. These 3 options represent increasing levels of complexity for implementation and maintenance. Hospitals with small and less-experienced informatics teams should be able to use the predesigned CDSTs that accompany hospital information systems. A "best practice alert" or some other types of notification are examples of these types of simple CDSTs. This type of alert may notify practitioners that a test order is a duplicate order, for example, customizing the activation of this type through minor modifications of the contents represents the next level of complexity. An example would be modifying an alert for a renally excreted drug so that it would only be activated if the drug order was placed for a patient with an estimated glomerular filtration rate below a certain threshold. Such an alert would be a tailored modification of an alert that otherwise would always alert the provider when that drug was being prescribed. This would be a mechanism to decrease the number of alerts seen by providers, and the modification makes it so that it is only activated when actually needed (ie, when the patient has decreased renal function). Finally, custom programming is required when desired intervention applications are not in the portfolio of the informatics vendor. The informatics team at the Cleveland Clinic has created or modified most of the interventions presented in this article in an effort to support our laboratory stewardship program. These include embedding data from recent laboratory tests within same-day duplicate test notifications, creating CDSTs that are activated for some providers but not others (ie, electronic privileging), creating alerts that are activated based on length of hospitalization, and creating alerts the fire based on the cost of the test being selected.[7–11]

Given these complexities, it has been our consistent recommendation to foster a strong and collaborative working relationship between the leadership of the laboratory stewardship committee and hospital informatics. This can be done in a variety of ways. A lead member of the hospital informatics team is a member for our laboratory stewardship committee. In this manner, she participates actively in the conversation and can experience firsthand the needs of the group or of the presenting provider. In addition, there is a standing meeting at our institution for the express purpose of monitoring the progress of projects that involve both pathology/laboratory medicine and hospital informatics. Although much of the meeting is devoted to the routine maintenance of the laboratory testing in a major medical center (ie, new test implementation, electronic public health reporting), a portion is devoted to tracking the building and implementation of test utilization initiatives.

PROJECT MANAGEMENT

There are several supporting elements for a test utilization program, the presence of which increase the likelihood of success. The importance of informatics support has already been emphasized. Important components of a successful test utilization or laboratory stewardship program includes active participation with genetic counselors, which is not covered in this article, project management, and the development and reporting of outcome measures, which is discussed below.

It will likely be difficult to convince hospital leadership to hire an individual to support a proposed laboratory stewardship program. Sometimes, as was the case in our institution, we needed to demonstrate effectiveness and cost-savings that could contribute toward the compensation of the project manager before being assigned such a resource. A full-time project manager is likely not needed, except, perhaps, in the largest and most robust of programs. Rather, the project manager could be a shared resource. Optimally, the task would be taken up by an individual who has signified or demonstrated interest in this area or a similar area, such as quality improvement or medical operations. Importantly, as laboratory stewardship management becomes another duty of that individual, in addition to the reason for their primary hire, it is important that they recognize that these are not secondary or optional assignments. To this end, there should be regular meetings between the project manager and the committee Chair(s) to review the progress of ongoing projects, discuss new projects, set the agenda of upcoming meetings, and any other miscellaneous work of the committee.

The committee Chair(s) is likely a busy physician, with limited time to perform all the necessary tasks for the organization and optimal management of the committee. Project managers are extremely effective in this manner.[3] They schedule meetings, assist with the formation and distribution of the meeting agenda, take and distribute minutes of meetings, and, possibly most importantly, interact with those involved regarding the progress on ongoing projects. The gentle pressure applied through regular and tactful prompting of responsible individuals is particularly important to move projects forward. Many projects will founder without this active management of the individual projects of the committee. Therefore, a project manager is extremely important, especially as the number of ongoing projects increases, because the Chair(s) will have limited capacity to manage these tasks in addition to his/her daily obligations.

OUTCOME MEASURES

It is not uncommon for individual, or groups of, physicians to make requests of the informatics department of a hospital to make changes, such as implementing CDS, that they believe will facilitate care delivery. It is also common that these changes are implemented without any follow-up with regard to the impact of the changes made. The use of CDSTs in modern medicine can irritate providers and hinder care delivery, even when thoughtfully vetted and implemented. Inconsiderate implementation of CDSTs without appropriate discovery, acquisition of clinical champions for the change, appropriate communications, and adequate ability to make rapid modifications should interventions function poorly is a recipe for failure. In addition to appropriately addressing the topics denoted above, the development of outcome reports is important.

It is important that someone or multiple individuals on the team have some expertise with data analysis, basic statistics, and report generation. The assessments of the impacts of test utilization initiatives should be factual with no inflation of the degree or meaningfulness of the impact. This inflation may not be intentional. For example, it is a common novice mistake to use charge information instead of actual cost information when determining the savings associated with an intervention. Charges represent the amount a provider would like to get paid for a service. The amount does not represent the cost of the service and rarely represents the amount actually paid for the service, given the variety of different payers. There is an excellent section Kent Lewandrowski's article, "Integrating Decision Support into a Laboratory Utilization Management Program,") in the Clinical and Laboratory Standards Institute's Developing and Managing a Medical Laboratory (Test) Utilization Management Program, which is recommended.[3]

Each of the interventions we describe below is associated with a unique monthly report that records the activity of each intervention. These reports are subsequently submitted to a dedicated financial officer who reviews and edits the reports for accuracy (ie, report scrubbing). Thereafter, a financial analysis is performed based on the costing and timing study data for each test for which there is a CDS intervention. A cost-savings report is then generated based on materials and labor savings. We have not sought to capture savings associated with stopping unnecessary phlebotomies or the stopping of other untoward events associated with poor test utilization.

These reports are collated annually to produce an annual report that demonstrates the efficacy of the interventions in our health care system (**Table 1**). Such a report is

Table 1
Project summary table

Project	Tests Avoided 2017	Cost-Savings 2017 ($)	Tests Avoided since Inception	Cost-Saving since Inception ($)	Lessons Learned
Best Practice Alert for Same-Day Duplicate Tests	N/A	N/A	N/A	N/A	A simple alert showed promise for highly specialized tests ordered by specialists, but was largely ignored for commonly ordered tests.
Hard Stops for Same-Day Duplicate Tests	4563	54,516	33,949	522,622	Communication with medical staff is essential. Consider a tiered implementation, beginning with a limited number of tests. A workaround is necessary, should the blockaded test be needed.
Extended Hard Stops	13,140	71,718	37,974	205,075	Extended hard stop interventions may help with C. *difficile* rates, and may provide insights into ordering patterns for the management of diabetes mellitus (eg, hemoglobin A1c frequencies).
Soft Stops for Same-Day Duplicate Tests	5507	41,258	26,767	211,800	The ability to override an electronic intervention at the computer order entry terminal will result in decreased compliance with the intervention compared with a hard stop intervention. This intervention, although less effective, still stops approximately half of the duplicate orders, and may be the only solution for settings unwilling to implement a hard stop.

Restricted Testing (Genetic Test Privileging)	57	67,262	565	1,094,659	Building and maintaining a list of privileged providers is an ongoing task. A workaround is necessary, should the blockaded test be needed.
Expensive Test Notifications	131	186,849	654	974,683	Chromosomal microarray studies and other molecular hematopathology tests constituted a large percentage of the tests averted by this intervention.
Three-Day Alerts for Stool Culture/Parasitologic Exams for Patients Hospitalized >3 Days	312	10,545	857	27,497	This intervention demonstrate the feasibility of implementing a classic intervention using an electronic format, which previously required intervention by a human.
Duplicate Constitutional Genetic Testing	350	45,183	940	132,743	Some requests for repeat testing were found to be valid, because exclusion codes were inadvertently not included in the programming (ie, codes to address QNS specimens, broken tubes)
Total	24,060	477,331	135,655	3,169,079	In addition to a substantial cost-savings, false-positive test results were avoided by not testing low-prevalence populations, which improves patient care, and the patient experience was enhanced by decreasing excessive phlebotomies and decreasing the cost of care.

The Best Practice Alert was used as a pilot. Although the number of tests averted was collected for pre-/post-comparison studies, this intervention was not retained.

Abbreviations: N/A, not applicable; QNS, quantity not sufficient for testing.

useful in a variety of ways. Foremost, the report should be shared with the leadership, who have supported the initiatives, and team members, who have brought the interventions to completion. The former demonstrates the competency of the group, which builds trust. The development of a reputation of a team that works for positive change within the institution in a collaborative way and accomplishes tasks will help secure future support. Sharing the annual report with team members provides an opportunity to genuinely thank them for their work and to demonstrate the larger view of the initiative to some who may have only seen their part of it. As more and more initiatives are added to the laboratory stewardship portfolio, analogies, and extrapolations can be made from previous experiences to new projects, which will facilitate implementation. Finally, although improvements in quality and patient care are the primary drivers of laboratory stewardship initiatives, the associated cost-savings are also important and should be reported. This savings should be collated for the projects implemented within the year, as well as year over year. Even initiatives with small savings add up over time. These cost-savings are appreciated by leadership and can also be used to garner support for new initiatives, and may be used to justify a new position (eg, project manager or genetics counselor).

EXAMPLES AND ASSOCIATED STUDIES

The Test Utilization Committee of the Cleveland Clinic, now re-branded as the laboratory stewardship committee, has been using CDSTs since 2011. Brief explanations and our experience with 8 CDS interventions, and any associated studies that have resulted from these projects follow.

Best Practice Alert for Same-Day Duplicate Tests

One of our earliest interventions at the Cleveland Clinic was using Best Practice Alerts or simple "Pop-up" notification for same-day duplicate testing. We first initiated this to study the effect of the intervention, with quantitative cytomegalovirus (CMV) testing and quantitative Epstein-Barr virus (EBV) testing. We selected these tests, because, through evidence, experience, and consensus between Infectious Diseases and Laboratory Medicine leadership, it was decided that same-day repeat testing for these viruses was not warranted.

The alert that was designed simply notified the provider that a same-day duplicate test was being ordered, and relied on the ordering provider to discontinue the order. We studied the same-day duplicate ordering of this test for 3 months before and 3 months after the intervention. To our pleasant surprise, there was a significant decrease in the number of duplicate orders placed after the intervention (data not shown; $P<.001$). We repeated the intervention in the same manner for same-day duplicate Clostridium difficile testing. To our unpleasant surprise, the results were opposite those we found for quantitative CMV and EBV testing. There was essentially no impact of the intervention for this test (data not shown; $P = .21$).

We have hypothesized on these stark differences. We believe, but did not definitively prove, that because quantitative CMV and EBV testing is usually only performed on a select group of patients by a select group of providers that the alert was read by, agreed to, and acted on appropriately. Conversely, because every intern, resident, and fellow in their busy day commonly consider the possibility of C difficile-associated diarrhea, the alert was likely ignored or, to use the colloquial "clicked through," and the duplicate order was placed. The reason for these differences remains conjecture, but we have subsequently performed timing studies regarding when the next order is placed after an electronic blockade, and have demonstrated that it is highly unlikely that the provider actually read the order (data not shown). Interestingly, Swimley and colleagues[12] demonstrated similar findings for *C difficile* testing, finding that, although some providers adhered to recommendations from the alert, the alert was often overridden resulting in no overall effect on *C difficile* testing rates.

These initiatives suggest that simple Best Practice Alerts or notifications may be used to curtail certain duplicate tests, possibly highly specialized tests ordered by highly specialized providers. These alerts are likely not regularly read and are less effective for commonly used tests; this behavior has been described for similar pharmacy-associated alerts.[13] This initiative provided our test utilization committee with the data needed to convince leadership to support the development of a hard stop for certain same-day duplicate tests.

Hard Stops for Same-Day Duplicate Tests

The introduction of the Same-Day Hard Stop CDST to avoid unnecessary same-day duplicate testing was undertaken in a tiered manner. This measured implementation was undertaken because this type of intervention (ie, a hard stop CDST) had never been used with providers at our institution. The leadership of our institution also required that we develop a mechanism by which the provider could obtain the test if they truly thought the duplicate test was medically necessary (ie, a bypass mechanism). We devised a process by which the ordering provider could work with our Laboratory Client Services, which is staffed 24/7, to place the desired order and effectively override the electronic blockade.

We began with a small number of tests that the test utilization committee agreed were not needed more than once per day. The list of 13 tests that were to be included in the Same-Day Hard Stop CDS trial was first shared with and approved by institutional leadership, and then shared with all medical staff via the hospital computer system. An opportunity for feedback concerning the tests on the list, as well as the initiative itself, was offered. One provider requested one of the tests to be removed, as he reported that, although rarely, he occasionally needed that particular test more than once per day in certain clinical scenarios. His request was granted, which reflected the philosophy of the test utilization committee of working to find areas of agreement and minimize academic arguments to move projects forward.

The Same-Day Hard Stop CDS was implemented for the 12 remaining tests, and to the surprise of many the implementation of the intervention was uneventful; requests to override the intervention, all of which were granted, were minimal. Therefore, the second tier of the rollout proceeded promptly, which included 77 additional tests; the addition of these tests was similarly uneventful. Finally, for the full-scale rollout, the physicians on the test utilization committee reviewed all tests on the test menu to determine which met the criteria of not being needed more than once per day. Only those for which there was consensus were targeted for inclusion. Over 1200 tests were included for the final phase of implementation of the Same-Day Hard Stop intervention.

Not surprisingly, there were a small number of instances wherein the subtleties of test use was not considered by the test utilization committee members. This occurred only 6 times and, in each instance, the provider requesting that a test be removed from the Same-Day Hard Stop list gave a valid reason. In addition, because of the excellent working relationship between the committee and the members of the hospital information technology group, the tests were able to be removed promptly (ie, within 24 hours). Feedback to the provider that their request had been heard and granted, and the test in question had been removed, helped team building with our clinical colleagues.

The details of the first 2 years of the Same-Day Hard Stop CDS intervention have been described previously.[9] Particularly interesting in this study was the documentation of the number of additional attempts to place the order after the electronic blockade was active, the language of which clearly stated that the provider needed to call Laboratory Client Services if they wanted to override the electronic blockade. This was interpreted as indirect evidence that the alert was not being read. In addition, the authors reviewed all the notifications of patient adverse events after the first year of implementation, and discovered no untoward events associated with this intervention. This finding, in conjunction with the fact that the provider was always given the right to override the intervention, brought the authors to the conclusion that this intervention was safe.

We reported that 11,790 unnecessary same-day duplicate test orders were prevented in the 2 years of this intervention, which saved the institution US$183,586 in materials and labor.[9] From 2011, when this intervention was implemented, through 2017, 33,949 unnecessary same-day duplicate test orders were stopped, saving the institution $522,622, and saving the patients a lot of unnecessary blood loss and pain.

Similarly, Dalal and colleagues[14] used a hard stop CDST to stop Free T3 (FT3) and Free T4 (FT4) orders placed on patients who had normal thyroid-stimulating hormone (TSH) levels. They reported a decrease in the ratio of FT4:TSH orders of 35.2% and a decreased FT3:TSH ratio of 55.2%. Furthermore, they found that the percentage of FT4 ordered due to abnormal TSH results increased by 126.1%. This intervention demonstrated a decrease in unnecessary testing, while increasing the appropriate use of the test. Hard stop CDSTs also have significant applications in the pharmacy domain to prevent dose-related patient safety issues.[15,16]

Extended Hard Stops

The success of the Same-Day Hard Stop CDST resulted in the recognition that some tests could be stopped for longer time periods. We initially examined an Extended Hard Stop CDST for hemoglobin A1c, hepatitis C genotyping, and C difficile testing. Hemoglobin A1c testing was limited to 30 days; it was recognized that this could be extended beyond 30 days, but, as previously stated, we favored achieving consensus and implementing the intervention, rather than risking a stalemate secondary to disagreements. Hepatitis C genotyping was slightly more controversial because of the recognized possibility of reinfection, but was retained because the same override mechanism as described above was in place. C difficile polymerase chain reaction testing was limited to one per week, and submitting stools for a test of cure was discouraged. This latter intervention has been useful in decreasing false-positives due to testing in a low-prevalence population (ie, individuals who have already tested negative). Others have also demonstrated the efficacy of using CDSTs as one of the tools to control inappropriate testing for C difficile.[17,18]

Subsequently, 30-day extended hard stops were added for 2 molecular hematopathology assays. Unlike the Same-Day Hard Stop CDST database, in which tests could be added or removed relatively easily, the addition of new tests for this intervention required an entirely new informatics build, which has significantly limited the ability to add new tests to this intervention. The Extended Hard Stop CDST was implemented at our institution in 2014. The process to override the electronic blockade from this CDST is the same as that described above. Since the implementation of the Extended Hard Stop CDST, this intervention has stopped 37,974 unnecessary tests and saved the institution $205,075.

Soft Stops for Same-Day Duplicate Tests

It was requested that we develop an intervention to address same-day duplicate testing at the regional hospitals of the Cleveland Clinic health system. There were several challenges that made the implementation of the Same-Day Hard Stop CDST unfeasible in the regional hospitals at that time. The intervention design consisted of an alert similar in configuration to that of the hard stop CDST, except that the ordering provider did not have to call Laboratory Client Services to override the intervention. The provider could simply bypass the electronic blockade at the point of computerized order entry and proceed with placing the order.

After implementation, we received and reviewed the monthly reports for the Soft Stop for Same-Day Duplicates at the regional hospitals. It became evident that the efficacy of the Soft Stop intervention was substantially less effective than the Same-Day Hard Stop CDST at the main campus. Therefore, we studied this intervention after a year and performed a comparison between the Same-Day Hard Stop CDST. This comparison is informative, because all of the tests that are on the Same-Day Soft Stop list are also on the Same-Day Hard Stop list. The Same-Day Hard Stop CDST was found to be 92.3% effective with respect to stopping the initially blockaded tests, whereas the Same-Day Soft Stop CDST was only 42.6% effective during the year in which both CDSTs were studied.[7] The cost-saving associated with the Same-Day Hard Stop CDST was $16.08/initial alert activation, whereas for the Same-Day Soft Stop CDST the saving was only $3.52/initial alert activation. These data demonstrated the superior efficacy and cost-savings associated with the Same-Day Hard Stop CDST compared with the Same-Day Soft Stop CDST. However, as noted above, there may be local issues that preclude the use of a hard stop CDST, so a soft stop may be the only option, which is better than no intervention.

The Soft Stop CDST for same-day duplicate tests has been in operation in our regional hospitals since 2013. It has stopped 26,767 unnecessary same-day duplicate orders and saved the institution $211,800.

Restricted Testing (Genetic Test Privileging)

Two initiatives were undertaken at the Cleveland Clinic to assure the appropriateness of molecular genetic test orders. These included the employment of a laboratory-based genetics counselor and the implementation of a Restricted Use CDST. Only the latter is discussed here, given the focus of this article, but the efficacy of both have been described.[10]

Our Restricted Use CDST intervention sought to limit molecular genetic testing to those individuals who used this testing routinely in their practice (ie, deemed users). We cited the precedent of limiting the use of certain therapeutic agents to certain groups of physicians (eg, certain antibiotics are restricted to infectious diseases practitioners and chemotherapy is largely limited to oncologists). Similarly, we explained to the leadership the great complexity of many of these assays, as well as the subtleties of these tests, which, if not appreciated during interpretation, pose a real possibility of misinterpretation and possible patient harm. These proved effective points to receive approval by senior leadership to move forward with this program.

Individuals who have received the Restricted Use CDST alert received language in the alert that notified them that if they believed the patient needed the molecular genetic test, then it could be obtained through a consultation with Medical Genetics or other deemed users. The implementation, apart from the construction of the deemed users list, was uneventful. Subsequently, we performed a focused review of patients for whom the Restricted Use CDST was activated. Three-quarters of inpatients for whom the Restricted Use CDST was activated did not receive a consultation, whereas for 25% a Medical Genetics consultation was placed. In the outpatient setting, the split was closer to 50:50. These data suggest that from 50% to 75% of the orders that were originally being placed by individuals not deemed to be experts in that area of testing (ie, not a deemed user) were not needed (ie, the ordering provider who was blocked did not obtain a consult). Conversely, we are pleased that between 25% and 50% of patients who may not have been scheduled to see an expert in the field necessary had a consult placed. The restricted use initiative was implemented in 2011, and although only 565 have been stopped by the Restricted Use CDST, these usually expensive tests have resulted in a cost-savings of $1,094,659.

A full assessment of CDS with respect to the diagnosis and management of patient with a genetic component to their health care issue is beyond the scope of this text. This field, however, is extensive. In addition to stopping unnecessary genetic testing, CDS has been used to more effectively guide providers in the optimal diagnosis and treatment of patients with a wide variety of diseases.[19–21]

Expensive Test Notifications

The listing of the cost of testing as a deterrent of excessive testing has been reviewed by several groups and the results are mixed. In our intervention, we decided to intervene for only the high-cost tests. We devised an alert that notified the provider that the test being ordered had a cost of $\geq$\$1000. This was initially done in \$1000 increments and then the range was expanded to include tests that cost $\geq$\$500. The language in the alert notified the provider that the charges of the tests exceed the cost and that charges not covered by insurance would be the responsibility of the patient. The intervention was not a hard stop, so the provider could bypass it and continue to place the order at the computer terminal without calling the laboratory.

We studied the efficacy of the Expensive Test CDST over a 3-year period.[11] The efficacy of this intervention was particularly interesting. If the absolute number of tests stopped by the Expensive Test CDST (ie, 654) was the indicator of success, then the intervention would be deemed ineffective, because only 12.5%, 12.9%, and 14.3% of the tests for which the CDST was activated were abandoned. However, if the cost-saving was the measure of the effectiveness of the intervention, then it would be considered successful, because the cost-savings for these 3 years was $696,007.

Sedrak and colleagues[22] undertook a randomized controlled trial examining the impact of displaying Medicare-allowable fees for inpatient tests. They found that displaying fees had no significant impact on overall clinician ordering behavior or associated fees. Schmidt and colleagues[23] also performed a randomized controlled trial to determine the impact of displaying the maximum Medicare reimbursement rate on test ordering behavior. This group, however, expanded the study to include both inpatients and outpatients, as well as different insurance categories (ie, government, commercial, and self-pay). They, like Sedrak, found that displaying this cost information had no impact on ordering behavior. Interestingly, they also assessed the charge awareness of residents and found that residents overestimated the charges of these tests. Horn and colleagues[24] studied the impact of the real-time cost display of the test commonly used by primary care physicians. In contrast to the previous 2 studies, they did find a significant relative decrease in 5 of the 21 tests for which the intervention was included. Considering that only 5 of the 21 tests were positively affected with respect to decreasing the ordering of laboratory tests, this group concluded that the real-time display of cost information could result in a modest reduction in laboratory testing.

Three-Day Alerts for Stool Culture/Parasitologic Examinations for Patients Hospitalized greater than 3 Days

There is a tenet in clinical microbiology that, for patients who have been hospitalized for greater than 3 days who develop diarrhea, that the diarrhea is not usually secondary to routine bacterial pathogens (ie, *Salmonella*, *Shigella*, *Campylobacter*, Enterohemorrhagic *E. coli*) or enteric parasites. Although there are recognized exceptions, for most individuals routine stool cultures or stool polymerase chain reaction, and ova and parasite examinations, are discouraged if diarrhea develops after 3 days of hospitalization.

We developed a CDST that determined the length of hospitalization at the time of order entry for stool culture and/or ova and parasite examinations. If the hospitalization was ≥3 days, then a hard stop alert was activated and the order could not be placed electronically. Similar to the Same-Day Hard Stop, the provider could override the electronic blockade, if they called Laboratory Client Services. We performed a pre-/post-analysis evaluating the ordering patterns for these tests 11 months before and after the implementation. After this intervention, there was a 54.1% reduction in ova and parasite microscopic morphologic examination ($P<.0001$), a 22.6% reduction in the *Giardia* and *Cryptosporidium* enzyme immunoassay ($P = .28$), and a 49.1% reduction in stool cultures ($P<.0001$).[8,25]

The cost-saving associated with this intervention is small, with only 857 unnecessary tests stopped since the implementation in 2014, with a cost-savings of $27,497. This serves as a reminder that these programs are about implementing best practices, rather than solely for the purpose of reducing health care costs.

Duplicate Constitutional Genetic Testing

It is recommended that genetic tests are not duplicated unless there is a good reason (eg, phenotype/genotype mismatch or concern over an erroneous result).[26] However, repeat constitutional genetic testing is not uncommon. We believe that this, in part, may be because of the unawareness of the practitioner that the test had previously been ordered, similar to our experience with the same-day duplicate hard stops. To address this issue, we devised a Duplicate Constitutional Genetic Test CDST, which placed a hard stop on any duplicate orders for 42 unique constitutional molecular genetic tests. As with previous interventions, the same procedure was used (ie, calling Laboratory Client Services) to override the electronic blockage, if the provider decided that a repeat test was medically necessary.

We studied the impact and efficacy of Duplicate Constitutional Genetic Test CDST over 3 years.[27] During this timeframe the CDST blocked 793 individual constitutional molecular genetic test orders; override requests were received and granted by Laboratory Client Services for 10.5% of the electronically blocked tests. A medical records review by our laboratory-based genetics counselor demonstrated that 81.9% of these were justified requests. Unfortunately, during the construction of this intervention, exclusion codes were not included for tests that were rejected for insufficient quantity of specimen, broken tube, and so forth. This resulted in justified override requests and has been remedied. The Duplicate Constitutional Genetic Test CDS intervention, which was implemented in 2015, has stopped 940 unnecessary tests and resulted in a $98,597 cost-savings for our institution. Similarly, Krasowski and colleagues[5] included duplicate alert notification in their overall strategy to improve test utilization.

SUMMARY

Although there have been substantial advances made in applications available in clinical information systems, additional progress is needed because most of the interventions described in this article required customized programming.[28,29] We have demonstrated the challenges and opportunities of operationalizing CDSTs of laboratory stewardship to improve medical care in a tertiary care medical center and the associated regional hospitals in our health system. The interventions described, as well as one not covered, which prevents excessive blood cultures, have, in aggregate, since their implementation, stopped 120,384 unnecessary tests and saved our institution $3,170,699.

Simple alerts are minimally effective and often not read because of alert fatigue and other factors. Hard stop CDSTs are more effective, but these must be used judiciously, so as to not interrupt care delivery. Furthermore, if these are used, a process by which the provider can bypass or override the alert should be developed. Current hospital information systems are lacking with respect to being able to provide advanced or custom CDSTs at present, so custom programming is necessary. Clinical decision support tools will remain a part of the hospital information system for the foreseeable future. When used carefully, these can assist in the appropriate delivery of care, while decreasing health care costs through the elimination of unnecessary testing and the sequelae thereof.

REFERENCES

1. Guo U, Chen L, Mehta PH. Electronic health record innovations: helping physicians - one less click at a time. Health Inf Manag 2017;46(3):140–4.
2. Dickerson JA, Fletcher AH, Procop G, et al. Transforming laboratory utilization review into laboratory stewardship: guidelines by the PLUGS National Committee for Laboratory Stewardship. J Appl Lab Med 2017;2(2):259–68.
3. Procop GW, Daley AT, Baron J, et al. GP49 developing and managing a medical laboratory (test) utilization management program. 1st edition. Wayne (PA): Clinical Laboratory Standards Institute; 2017.
4. Elwyn G, Scholl I, Tietbohl C, et al. "Many miles to go ...": a systematic review of the implementation of patient decision support interventions into routine clinical practice. BMC Med Inform Decis Mak 2013;13(Suppl 2):S14.
5. Krasowski MD, Chudzik D, Dolezal A, et al. Promoting improved utilization of laboratory testing through changes in an electronic medical record: experience at an academic medical center. BMC Med Inform Decis Mak 2015;15:11.
6. Wilson ML. Decreasing inappropriate laboratory test utilization: controlling costs and improving quality of care. Am J Clin Pathol 2015;143(5):614–6.
7. Procop GW, Keating C, Stagno P, et al. Reducing duplicate testing: a comparison of two clinical decision support tools. Am J Clin Pathol 2015;143(5):623–6.
8. Procop GW, Nikolic D, Asamoto K, et al. Reply to Beal et al., 'The "3-Day Rule" for stool tests may not apply when using PCR panels. J Clin Microbiol 2018;56(4).
9. Procop GW, Yerian LM, Wyllie R, et al. Duplicate laboratory test reduction using a clinical decision support tool. Am J Clin Pathol 2014;141(5):718–23.
10. Riley JD, Procop GW, Kottke-Marchant K, et al. Improving molecular genetic test utilization through order restriction, test review, and guidance. J Mol Diagn 2015;17(3):225–9.
11. Riley JD, Stanley G, Wyllie R, et al. The impact of an electronic expensive test notification. Am J Clin Pathol 2018;149(6):530–5.
12. Swimley K, Olsen R, Long SW, et al. Failure of best practice alerts to affect C. difficile test utilization. Am J Clin Pathol 2018;150:S143–68.
13. Cho I, Lee Y, Lee JH, et al. Wide variation and patterns of physicians' responses to drug-drug interaction alerts. Int J Qual Health Care 2018. https://doi.org/10.1093/intqhc/mzy102.
14. Dalal S, Bhesania S, Silber S, et al. Use of electronic clinical decision support and hard stops to decrease unnecessary thyroid function testing. BMJ Qual Improv Rep 2017;6(1) [pii:u223041.w8346].

15. Grissinger M. Small effort, big payoff: automated maximum dose alerts with hard stops. P T 2016;41(2):82–128.
16. Martin DB, Kaemingk D, Frieze D, et al. Safe implementation of computerized provider order entry for adult oncology. Appl Clin Inform 2015;6(4):638–49.
17. Friedland AE, Brown S, Glick DR, et al. Use of computerized clinical decision support for diagnostic stewardship in *Clostridioides difficile* testing: an academic hospital quasi-experimental study. J Gen Intern Med 2018;34(1):31–2.
18. Madden GR, German Mesner I, Cox HL, et al. Reduced *Clostridium difficile* tests and laboratory-identified events with a computerized clinical decision support tool and financial incentive. Infect Control Hosp Epidemiol 2018;39(6):737–40.
19. Freimuth RR, Formea CM, Hoffman JM, et al. Implementing genomic clinical decision support for drug-based precision medicine. CPT Pharmacometrics Syst Pharmacol 2017;6(3):153–5.
20. Graham MM, James MT, Spertus JA. Decision support tools: realizing the potential to improve quality of care. Can J Cardiol 2018;34(7):821–6.
21. Hasnie AA, Kumbamu A, Safarova MS, et al. A clinical decision support tool for familial hypercholesterolemia based on physician input. Mayo Clin Proc Innov Qual Outcomes 2018;2(2):103–12.
22. Sedrak MS, Myers JS, Small DS, et al. Effect of a price transparency intervention in the electronic health record on clinician ordering of inpatient laboratory tests: the PRICE randomized clinical trial. JAMA Intern Med 2017;177(7):939–45.
23. Schmidt RL, Colbert-Getz JM, Milne CK, et al. Impact of laboratory charge display within the electronic health record across an entire academic medical center: results of a randomized controlled trial. Am J Clin Pathol 2017;148(6): 513–22.
24. Horn DM, Koplan KE, Senese MD, et al. The impact of cost displays on primary care physician laboratory test ordering. J Gen Intern Med 2014;29(5):708–14.
25. Nikolic D, Richter SS, Asamoto K, et al. Implementation of a clinical decision support tool for stool cultures and parasitological studies in hospitalized patients. J Clin Microbiol 2017;55(12):3350–4.
26. Choosing wisely: smart decisions about genetic testing. 2015. Available at: http://www.choosingwisely.org/patient-resources/making-smart-decisions-about-genetic-testing/. Accessed October 12, 2018.
27. Riley JD, Stanley G, Wyllie R, et al. An electronic strategy to eliminate duplicate genetic testing using clinical decision support (Poster No. 152). CAP18 The Pathologists' Meeting. October 20–24, 2018. Chicago, IL.
28. Islam MM, Poly TN, Li YJ. Recent advancement of clinical information systems: opportunities and challenges. Yearb Med Inform 2018;27(1):83–90.
29. Rubinstein M, Hirsch R, Bandyopadhyay K, et al. Effectiveness of practices to support appropriate laboratory test utilization: a laboratory medicine best practices systematic review and meta-analysis. Am J Clin Pathol 2018;149(3): 197–221.

Decision Support and Patient Safety

Mario Plebani, MD, FRCP[a,b,*], Ada Aita, PhD[a,b], Andrea Padoan, PhD[a,b], Laura Sciacovelli, MSc[c]

KEYWORDS

- Clinical decision support • Health IT • Laboratory reports • Critical results
- Quality indicators

KEY POINTS

- CDS systems not only support IT, but also enable the exchange of all available information, thus helping clinicians make the best possible decision.
- CDS systems, in a wide sense, are "any other knowledge-driven interventions that can promote safety, education, workflow improvement, communication, and improved quality of care."
- Web-based supports can be used as tools to meet clinicians' and patients' needs by enhancing links between them, and to measure and improve quality performance.
- Quality measurement and reporting represent a form of CDS; health IT should be the means by which evidence is developed to support decision-making.
- Assistive information included in laboratory reports can support the right interpretation of results in making a diagnosis or designing a personalized treatment plan.

INTRODUCTION

Laboratory testing, which is multifaceted and referred to as the total testing process (TTP), includes several steps, from selection of laboratory tests to the release of test results to requesting physicians. In the last few years, a body of evidence has been collected to demonstrate the strategic role of laboratory information in relation to the action undertaken to the patient, and the association between laboratory tests and further diagnostic or therapeutic interventions. Lundberg,[1] who emphasized the importance of the relationship between all stakeholders, above all, clinicians and

Disclosure Statement: The authors have nothing to disclose.
[a] Department of Laboratory Medicine, University-Hospital of Padova, via Giustiniani 2, Padova 35128, Italy; [b] Department of Medicine - DIMED, University of Padova, via Giustiniani 2, Padova 35128, Italy; [c] Department of Laboratory Medicine, University-Hospital of Padova, via Giustiniani 2, Padova 35128, Italy
* Corresponding author. Department of Laboratory Medicine, University-Hospital of Padova, via Giustiniani 2, Padova 35128, Italy.
E-mail address: mario.plebani@unipd.it

Clin Lab Med 39 (2019) 231–244
https://doi.org/10.1016/j.cll.2019.01.003
labmed.theclinics.com

laboratorians, stated that they "should all be concerned about the effects of that laboratory test and whether the performance of it was useful for the patient or for the public's health," thus stressing the need for research into outcomes. It is therefore essential to ensure that appropriate information is adequately defined and effectively interpreted.[2] In this context, the promotion and development of clinical decision support (CDS) systems, focusing on all TTP activities, can help to guarantee the effective communication of all strategic information between all involved stakeholders, facilitate error prevention and improve patient care provision.

Scientific literature dealing with CDS has focused on the use of information technology (IT), such as health care information systems (HIS), laboratory information systems (LIS), and specific computerized and Web-based applications.[3] However, some investigators, such as Osheroff[4] and Shoolin,[5] underline that CDS should not be interpreted only as a tool providing information support or rules and algorithms, but rather as a system allowing the exchange and use of all information, thus helping clinicians make the best possible decision by considering all quality aspects involved in the enhancement of performance. Teich and colleagues[6] report that CDS systems, in a wider sense, are "any other knowledge-driven interventions that can promote safety, education, workflow improvement, communication, and improved quality of care."

In view of the above, CDS applied to Laboratory Medicine refers to all information, adequately structured and realized in an accurate and timely way, and also provided by and transferred to the right person within the framework of an appropriate control process. According to the Agency for Healthcare Research and Quality, improvements in desired health care outcome using CDS systems and strategies can be achieved by following the CDS Five rights approach, which includes the need to communicate:

1. The *right information*, evidence-based, suitable for guiding clinical actions, pertinent to the circumstance
2. To the *right person*, considering all stakeholders (eg, staff, clinicians, patients, citizens)
3. In the *right CDS intervention format*, such as an alert, order set, or reference information to answer a clinical question
4. Through the *right channel*, for example, an information system such as an electronic medical record (EMR), LIS, or a more general channel such as the Internet or a mobile device
5. At the *right time in workflow*, for example, at time of decision/action/need[7]

The use of this approach in Laboratory Medicine in each phase of the TTP, not only in laboratory test selection and results interpretation where it has usually been applied, allows operators to ensure that every activity is carried out with optimal effectiveness, safety, and resource use.[4,5,8–10]

INFORMATION RESOURCES IN CDS

The disappointing data published in the Institute of Medicine report *To Err Is Human*[11,12] prompted the proposal to use informatics in order to make health care processes safer. Bar coding, computerized physician order entry, crew resource management, and simulators have been considered possible strategies for identifying and reducing errors attributed mainly to cognitive factors and handoff, but also to system failures. However, health IT should not be thought of as a single product, but as a technical system that works in a larger sociotechnical system including people, processes, organization, and the external environment (eg, regulations). Its design, should therefore take into account all sociotechnical components. Although studies focusing on health IT and patient safety are complex and subject to methodological bias, it has been observed that health IT has a negative affect when it: alters the workflow or is poorly integrated into it[13]; is not user-friendly[14] or reliable[15]; continues to use both paper and electronic-based systems.[13] However, on reviewing literature on the impact of health IT in each phase of the laboratory TTP in primary care, Maillet and colleagues[16] found that most studies report that IT makes an important contribution to TTP, enhancing its efficiency, reliability, and timeliness.

In recent years, the use of IT systems has greatly increased in laboratories, thus facilitating the management of all activities, meeting clinicians' and patients' needs by creating efficient links between them and measuring and improving performance quality.[17] Many integrated health care delivery systems use information systems and integrated decision support to manage quality assurance activities and to ensure excellent performance.[18] The integration of electronic systems such as HIS, LIS, middleware, or specifically designed software, in conjunction with skilled and knowledgeable staff, crucial to the promotion of data quality, guarantees the traceability of data and activities, ensures uniformity of policy and practice, and completeness with data accuracy. By using highly flexible applications and programming interfaces the laboratory can improve on the use of information inside and outside the laboratory, thus enhancing hospital and health care. Numerous investigators have highlighted the improvements achieved in Laboratory Medicine through the use of dedicated software and stressed the role of laboratory professionals in this field, recognizing the development of informatics as a sub-specialty within the discipline of Laboratory Medicine.[19–24]

APPLICATION AND OPPORTUNITIES FOR CDS IN LABORATORY MEDICINE

Although, there is no consensus on the features of IT constituting CDS, these systems can be implemented using a variety of platforms (eg, Internet-based, local personal computer, networked EMR, or a handheld device) as well as a variety of computing approaches. However, commonly used CDS systems include the divulgation of knowledge, programs for combining the knowledge with patient-specific information, and communication mechanisms. The assessment and improvement of TTP quality, cost saving, and technical/organizational integration are critical to the effective management of information, enhancing patient safety and raising awareness of the role and importance of laboratories within health care organizations.[25,26] By using appropriate CDS, laboratories can provide value-added features, fill the knowledge gaps among clinicians, supervise testing according to recommended guidelines, and provide increasingly efficient and cost-effective testing.[27] According to a recently published meta-analysis, computerized provider order entry and CDS systems are effective tools for improving appropriateness in test requesting, particularly when used in association with education practice.[28]

In Laboratory Medicine, CDS encompasses a variety of tools including: computerized alerts and reminders for providers and patients; clinical guidelines; condition/disease-specific order set; patient-oriented reports and summaries; documentation templates; diagnostic support; contextually relevant reference information.[4] Laboratories have implemented computerized applications, using Microsoft (Microsoft, Redmond, WA, USA) tools such as Access and Excel to automate all possible steps of TTP. In parallel, vendors have begun to produce and commercialize laboratory software packages to be integrated with HIS and LIS. This indicates an increasingly pressing need for new software packages that interface with LIS and other information systems to extract data in a standardized way, so as to detect laboratory errors, facilitate analysis, and improve laboratory quality management and resource use.

Systems for Sharing Laboratory Test Information

The increased complexity of laboratory tests coupled with ever more sophisticated technologies and greater precision medicine, calls for laboratory professionals to actively help clinicians correctly manage laboratory tests, assist patients and citizens, and provide all necessary information on aspects that can impact on suitability of results. In this context, Web-based laboratory handbooks could easily be implemented and shared with all the involved stakeholders. Web-based handbooks should contain all necessary information on tests and their clinical utility, and also provide basic interpretative advice, specifying any interferences, possible causes of false-positive and false-negative results. Moreover, information such as collection instructions, turnaround time (TAT), and cost, can be an efficient tool for maintaining, updating and sharing laboratory information, contributing to and guaranteeing the reliability of laboratory results, and favoring sound clinical decision-making.[17]

Our laboratory has developed an online laboratory handbook (**Fig. 1**), the so-called "logbook," in which all tests provided by the laboratory are listed; **Table 1** shows the information provided for each test. Access to information is controlled according to the type of user. Laboratory staff can visualize all information included in the logbook, whereas other health care personnel (requesters), such as clinicians of other laboratories using the laboratory service, can visualize all information useful for an adequate collection of blood or other biological material and interpretation of results (eg, possible error cause or interference, or measurement uncertainty). Patients and citizens, on the other hand, only have access to general information explaining whether or not the laboratory provides the service they are interested in and, if so, the time it takes to report the result.

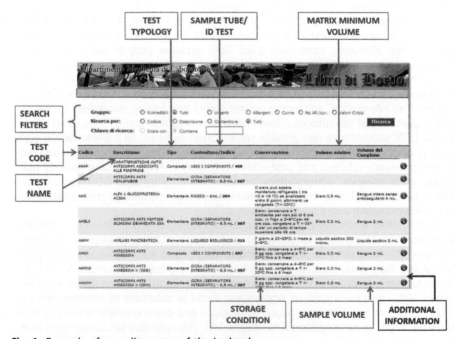

Fig. 1. Example of an online page of the logbook.

Table 1

Information reported in the Logbook of the Department of Laboratory Medicine of the University Hospital of Padova (Italy) and visualizable by the different users.

Information	Laboratory / Laboratory Intranet	Laboratory + Other Requesters (Clinicians, Other Laboratories) / Hospital Intranet	Patients and Citizens / Web	Information Extraction
Name of test, synonyms and identification code	X	X	X	LIS
Type of matrix required, with related volume, and container (for test tube, cap color also indicated)	X	X	X	LIS
Storage and treatment immediately after collection	X	X	X	Manual entry
Measurement units	X	X	X	LIS
Reference intervals or/and decisional levels (RI/DL)	X	X	X	LIS
Origin and date of last RI/DL revision	X	—	—	Manual entry
Scope of test and/or clinical information (significance of increased or decreased values)	X	X	X	Manual entry
Interferences and possible error cause	X	X	X	Manual entry
Determination method	X	—	—	Manual entry
Type of method (IVD or in-house)	X	—	—	Manual entry
Measurement uncertainty (MU) and/or total error allowable (TEa) and/or RCV and date of their last revision	X	Only on request	—	LIS
Availability of IQC and EQA	X	—	—	Manual entry
EQA provider	X	—	—	Manual entry
Reporting time	X	X	X	LIS
Cost	X	X	X	LIS
Section of laboratory where test is determined and person in charge?	X	X	—	Manual entry

Abbreviations: EQA, external quality assessment; IQC, internal quality control; IVD, in vitro diagnostic.

An information support process extracts all testing information included in the LIS and structures the data in an easily understandable form that allows a speedy search to be made using, for example, the test name, its code, and/or synonym. The extraction from LIS guarantees information accuracy and prevents errors due to data entry and the congruity of data reported in more than 1 document or place when updating is needed. Unfortunately, not all information is included in the LIS, with manual input being required for the non-included data. The laboratory handbook combines information contained in several support systems (computerized or paper documents) to facilitate the update process, or for other reasons such as document printing. A laboratory Web site grouping together all the support systems used is an effective tool and is increasingly widely used in the context of health care.

An access-restricted private subnetwork (Intranet) can be used in many other activities involved in the management of quality aspects. It can, for example, contain a centralized repository of laboratory documentation concerning laboratory policy, criteria, processes, procedures, and instructions. The advantage of keeping documentation online in a private network is that its log-in system guarantees distribution exclusively to personnel with authorized access, obviates the use of obsolete documentation, tracks access, and ensures that all documentation needed is issued. Likewise, an intranet network can be used to collect data in a repository that is accessible at all times to each area of laboratory, whether simultaneously or at different times, to several authorized staff members. The collection and registration of undesirable events (eg, errors, inadequate samples, delayed TAT) occurring during the routine flow appear in a shared support system, thus raising awareness of potential problems, promoting communication between interested parties and encouraging the staff in charge of their resolution to assume responsibility.

Management of Quality Indicators

In the last 20 years, along with the growing awareness of the importance of quality and safety in health care, quality assessment has also become crucial to promoting informed decision-making and safe and reliable care through monitoring, analyzing, and communicating the degree to which health care organizations meet key goals. The identification of reliable quality indicators (QIs) in the TTP is an important step in the quality assessment process because it enables all stakeholders to quantify the quality of selected laboratory service domains.[29,30] A QI is thus intended as "an objective measure that potentially evaluates all critical care domains as defined by the IOM (patient safety, effectiveness, equity, patient-centeredness, timeliness and efficiency), that is based on evidence associated with those domains, and can be implemented in a consistent and comparable manner across settings and over time."[31]

However, QIs alone do not directly improve performance and guarantee patient safety, but act as alerts or flags, drawing the attention of users to areas that need improvement or more detailed investigation.[32] Essential tools for individual laboratories allowing the internal identification of high-risk processes and procedures, they can also be used as external benchmarks for identifying and testing the level of structure, process, and outcome quality among laboratories.[30,33] A practical application of QIs as a tool to guarantee patient safety has been presented by Flegar-Meštric and colleagues.[34] Aiming to reduce errors occurring in pre-analytical processes in an emergency department with the highest rate of errors, the investigators performed a risk analysis by using data from 22 harmonized QIs and, by quantifying risk, they prioritized actions toward process components most in need of improvement to reduce the patient risks to clinically acceptable levels. Regular tailored education, as well as standardization and computerization of processes (eg, identification of samples, distribution of educational materials and protocols), were identified as corrective and preventive actions after data analysis and led to a reduction in pre-analytical errors in the emergency laboratory, thus enhancing patient safety and health care outcomes.[34]

The awareness that undesirable outcomes are generally the result of unrecognized and/or unmanaged risk, has prompted widespread efforts to use collected patient and sample data to identify quality measures and provide feedback to clinicians. However, the efficacy of monitoring performance strictly depends on: (a) the completeness and quality of information collected; (b) the metric and targets identified to assess the success of utilization management strategies.[35] The development of QIs calls, above all, for expertise of laboratory professionals who can identify the set of unambiguous and statistically sound measures, addressing all stages of the TTP and focused on areas pertinent to the needs of users (patient safety, quality, and cost-effective process). To this end, several QI programs have been launched in different countries (eg, Royal College of Pathologists Australasia, Quality Assurance Programs, Key Incident Monitoring and Management System, College of American Pathologists Q-Tracks, Brazilian Laboratory Indicators).[36–40] However, these institutions have included measures that differ in number, type, terminology, and target used, thus complicating benchmarking of processes. Only recently, thanks to laboratory professionals, and under the umbrella of the International Federation of Clinical Chemistry and Laboratory Medicine, has general consensus been achieved on a standardized set of QIs, known as Model of Quality Indicators, reliable for number, type, terminology, rationale, purpose, collection method, target setting, and information to report to participating laboratories.[41]

The standardization and harmonization of QI data recording are still challenging issues. To guarantee quality of data and minimize any burden on time and resources, data should be collected as part of a coherent and integrated system in routine service delivery. A robust IT environment that can guarantee standardization, accuracy, and efficacy of data collection is fundamental to achieving this. Several years ago, a pre-analytical error recording software based on Microsoft Access was developed for standardizing data collection and called for users to record the date of specimen receipt, sample ID, patient name, type of request, referring ward, sample matrix, type of non-conformity, action undertaken to solve the problem, possible additional actions undertaken, and the operator's personal code.[42] In 2017, this program was updated and standardized according to the most recent Federation of Clinical Chemistry and Laboratory Medicine Model of Quality Indicator review.[43] Our laboratory now uses a recently introduced computerized application for the daily recording of all undesirable TTP events (including information such as error type, patient identification details, sample type and source, required tests, recording operators) that are processed for statistical analysis. With this application, staff members use an appropriate device to scan the barcode of an unsuitable sample (eg, hemolyzed, clotted, insufficient), and the output information is automatically relayed to a computer and structured in tabular form. This process, which allows the easy extraction and export onto spreadsheets of all recorded data, generates rapid and efficient local statistics to be used to track errors and establish proactive strategies for their prevention.[30,43]

Other types of error, concerning requests, results, medical reports, unsatisfactory performance in External Quality Assessment Scheme, are managed in a similar way. All information on each request or sample is automatically recorded with, in particular, the patient's ID details and the area where the request was received (eg, name and surname of patient, identification code [ID], type of request), the sample collected (eg, sample number or origin of the specimen, sample matrix).[30] This application also allows visualization of data trends over time, simplifies data analysis, and is conducive to establishing proactive strategies for the prevention of errors based on the best available information.[30,33] In this context, if one of the purposes of CDS is to improve quality and safety of care processes, then quality measurement and reporting represents a passive form of CDS, and health IT, being the means by which evidence is developed in order to support decision-making.

Notification of Critical Results

The notification of critical laboratory results in as short a time possible, is a laboratory activity that strongly impacts on patients outcome. To ensure effective communication of critical results, the following must be guaranteed:

- Identification of analytes that, at defined concentration levels, highlight a critical health condition for patients
- Prompt notification by laboratory professionals
- Cognizant reception of communication by physicians in charge of patients
- Compliance with privacy laws and traceability needs

Lundberg defined critical laboratory results as "a value that represents a pathophysiological state at such variance with normal that prompt medical intervention is required to avert imminent danger for the patient concerned, and for which effective action is possible."[44] Before the implementation of a quality management system complying with International Standard requirements, all necessary steps were carried out by involved professionals, but without evidence of these steps being taken by authorized staff, at specified times and in accordance with defined procedures. Moreover, all activities were kept under control with the use of paper documentation; but, now, with dedicated electronic support we can achieve high levels of assurance of effectiveness and traceability.

Piva, Plebani and colleagues,[45,46] described a management of a critical results system based on the:

- Clear definition of critical values
- Identification of responsibilities
- Implementation of electronic notification systems

The electronic notification system/automatically sends a short message (SMS) generated by HIS as soon as values have been validated by the clinical pathologist in charge in the LIS and fed into the HIS. The message text, sent to the cell phone of the referring physician,[47,48] reports the critical result using the patient's ID code but, for reasons of privacy in the case of inpatients, the physician is invited to access HIS for the consultation of patient details and related critical results, whereas GPs are asked to urgently contact the laboratory. Furthermore, all the steps of the process are recorded in the electronic platform: critical results identified, the sending of the SMS, the visualization of the result by physician or the contact received by family doctor, and all related times. The laboratory is responsible for the appropriate TAT, including the time in which the result is effectively reported to the clinician, so that the recording system allows all times to be monitored, in particular: the TAT of testing (from sample reception to release of result) and the time from availability of result to the reception of laboratory information by physician or family doctor.

An electronic process has numerous advantages over a manual one because it guarantees the control of all phases of the specific process and creates significant time-savings, as well as the possibility for statistical evaluations, which are crucial to identifying improvement opportunities. Moreover, an electronic system ensures accuracy of recording, of crucial importance, as recorded data are an important source for QIs.[30,32] Software for the management of critical results should be made available to laboratories worldwide to promote harmonization of procedures and practices and assure the quality and safety in laboratory testing.[49]

Information in Laboratory Reports

The International Standard ISO 15189:2012,[50] concerning the reporting of laboratory results (par. 5.8), requires that "*The results of each examination shall be reported accurately, clearly, unambiguously and in accordance with any specific instructions in the examination procedures. .... Reports shall include the information necessary for the interpretation of the examination results.*"

Laboratory reports are known to include not only test results, but also further crucial additional information that can be effectively used for clinical decision-making. However, the effectiveness of information provided by laboratories in their reports strictly depends on the typologies of the parameters included, the level of their quality and the clarity of their arrangement. During the last few decades, in addition to the examination results reported in SI units, units traceable to SI units or other applicable units and compared with reference intervals (RIs), laboratory professionals have included further parameters in reports to support the clinician's interpretation of test results, including, in particular, previous results of the same patient with reference change value (RCV); flagging to highlight results (outside RI or critical) for prompt consideration; information on analytical variability that may affect the result; interpretative comments and diagnostic algorithms.

The RI and/or decisional limit (DL) is indispensable for guaranteeing interpretation of results in relation to technology used, demographic characteristics of population or clinical context, and patient features (eg, sex, age, pathophysiological condition). Comparing a patient's result with the corresponding RI/DL is the main procedure used by the clinician to evaluate the patient's condition. The appropriate definition of RI/DL, and its periodic revision, is therefore crucial to providing the right information and preventing post-analytical errors that lead to incorrect interpretation and use of laboratory results.[51,52]

Another procedure used for interpretation of test results includes the comparison between 2 sequential results for a specific analyte. When the observed variation, including variation associated with the examination procedure as well as inherent biological variation, exceeds the defined RCV, a significant change has occurred. The formula defining the appropriate RCV is established, together with all possible conditions that can affect the reliability of the comparison made. Laboratory professionals provide RCV for analytes where this parameter is useful for diagnostic purposes, for monitoring a patient, and for suggesting, or changing, a treatment. As this parameter takes into account 2 sequential results from the same individual, it is mainly used to obtain a more objective interpretation of a measured difference found in patient monitoring.[53] Analytical measurement error, like total error, cannot be completely eliminated and should be taken into account in the results interpretation. These 2 sources of error, systematic and random,[54] should be within acceptable limits in order not to affect interpretation suitability.

The recent estimation of error measurement, which is the measurement uncertainty (MU), has been endorsed by the ISO15189:2012.[50] Although debate on how to use this value inside and outside the laboratory is ongoing, a proposal for the inclusion of MU in laboratory reports has recently been developed, as follows: (a) when a test result is usually compared with RI, MU should be included in the laboratory report as a confidence interval given at a defined confidence level (eg, 95%), calculated using only the component of laboratory imprecision; (b) when a test result is compared with a clinical decision point (eg, cut-off, decision limit, and/or critical value), the MU should be calculated by including not only imprecision but also bias; (c) when a test result is used for monitoring a disease and or/therapy, the RCV is the most appropriate information to provide.[51,55] In all cases, the communication of MU for supporting clinical decision-making calls for strong involvement of laboratory professionals in terms of technical and communication skills.

Furthermore, the complexity of laboratory diagnostics has increased the need to include interpretative advice in laboratory reports. Medical laboratories may offer advice on test interpretation as well as on further appropriate investigation. The type of interpretative comments provided in the reports may vary in depth because of the degree of individualization and may depend not only on the complexity of the test, but also on the requesting clinician and the expertise available within the laboratory.[56]

The competency of laboratory professionals in the formulation of consistent and correct interpretative comments, combined with communication skills, is therefore of utmost importance in supporting clinicians in their decision-making. However, as the formulation of interpretative comments can require a different specificity depending on each clinical case, comments from different professionals may differ, although they are addressed to provide the same indication (eg, probable diagnosis; diagnosis that can be ruled out; additional investigation). Consequently, clinicians can save time in the interpretation and use of information provided in laboratory reports if the formulation complies with harmonized criteria.[57] Recently, an example of harmonization of the interpretative comments in hematology has been proposed.[58]

Several tools are implemented in the laboratory to control the suitability of the interpretative comments provided; the competence of professionals in charge of formulating them and the congruity of comments provided by different professionals concerning the same clinical case (eg, participation in External Quality Assessment Schemes; implementation of internal surveys, codification of predefined comments).[57,59] Therefore, as interpretive comments are considered a fundamental CDS in patient management, laboratory professionals have an important role. Because interpretative comments can be an effective CDS tool, laboratory professionals must ensure that they are appropriate and harmonized.

Another aspect that impacts on the user-friendliness of laboratory information is the way in which it is arranged in the report. On conducting a survey to evaluate the formatting of laboratory reports used in several Australian laboratories for some numerical biochemistry results, the Royal College of Pathologists of Australasia[60] found a wide variability due to many inter-laboratory differences including the following: test names for the same measurand, units, and RIs, decimal places to report results and RIs, results flagging mode, alignment of results, and formatting of different components in the reports. Although these items might seem insignificant against the importance of accuracy of results, it must be borne in mind that clear and consistent reporting, complying with approved guidelines, has a strong impact on patient safety. It has been demonstrated that the understanding of laboratory information depends largely on the formatting choices that are not only time saving, but also allow the user to speedily grasp key information. Moreover, the adherence to approved guidelines guarantees harmonization among different laboratories, thus facilitating the clinician's activity.[60]

Formatting, as well as additional parameters in laboratory reports (some of which are described above) for supporting and enhancing the clinical decision, can be well managed by the use of informatics, not only for electronic generation of reports and long-term storage, as required by law. In particular, the LIS should interface with other information systems, thus providing additional relevant information, such as that contained in the patient's EMR or the parameters related to the test used (eg, contained in the laboratory log book). This intertwined system can allow, for example, the calculation of gender- and age-specific RI, but also the prompt inclusion in reports of, among other items, RCV, MU, and previous results. In this way, support for the right interpretation coupled with other helpful information on the patient effectively gives the ordering physician the opportunity to review the laboratory tests results thoroughly, before making a diagnosis or designing a personalized treatment plan.

SUMMARY

Quality in laboratory testing must be guaranteed in all steps of the so-called "Brain-to-brain loop," from the "pre-pre-analytical" phase ("Right test choice at the Right time on the Right patient"), through the analytical steps ("Right results in the Right forms"), and on to the "post-post-analytical" phase ("Right interpretation, at the Right time with the Right advice as to what to do next with the result").[2,61,62] Clinical laboratory stewardship seems to be an effective tool in achieving this goal, by promoting interaction and cooperation between clinicians and laboratory professionals from the first to the final steps of the total testing process.[62] Given the increasing complexity of laboratory tests, the active support of laboratory professionals is the key to the provision of support for clinicians, who need to correctly manage laboratory test results to maximize patient safety.

The development and sharing of CDS has been invaluable in disseminating and implementing evidence-based knowledge into clinical practice, and engaging stakeholders, including laboratory professionals, clinicians and family doctors, and health IT vendors, as well as patients and citizens. CDS systems, are not only information and communication technologies, but are, above all, educational initiatives giving users and providers feedback, expert consultation activated at each stage of the TTP, and have proved to be extremely useful tools in assuring performance quality and helping clinicians make the best possible decision for each and every patient.

REFERENCES

1. Lundberg GD. The need for an outcomes research agenda for clinical laboratory testing. JAMA 1998;280:565–6.
2. Plebani M, Laposata M, Lundberg GD. The brain-to-brain loop concept for laboratory testing 40 years after its introduction. Am J Clin Pathol 2011;136:829–33.
3. Beeler PE, Bates DW, Hug BL. Clinical decision support systems. Swiss Med Wkly 2014;144:w14073.
4. Osheroff JA, Teich JM, Middleton B, et al. A roadmap for national action on clinical decision support. J Am Med Inform Assoc 2007;14:141–5 [Erratum in: J Am Med Inform Assoc 2007;14:389].
5. Shoolin JS. Clinical decision support and the electronic health record-applications for physiatry. PM R 2017;9:S34–40.
6. Teich JM, Osheroff JA, Pifer EA, et al, CDS Expert Review Panel. Clinical decision support in electronic prescribing: recommendations and an action plan: report of the joint clinical decision support workgroup. J Am Med Inform Assoc 2005;12: 365–76.
7. Eichner J, Das M. Challenges and barriers to clinical decision support (CDS) design and implementation experienced in the agency for healthcare research

and quality CDS demonstrations. Rockville (MD): Agency for Healthcare Research and Quality; 2010. AHRQ Publication No. 10-0064-EF.

8. Agency for Healthcare Research and Quality (AHRQ). Health Information Technology best-practices transforming quality, safety, and efficiency. Available at: https://healthit.ahrq.gov/ahrq-funded-projects/current-health-it-priorities/clinical-decision-support-cds/chapter-1-approaching-clinical-decision/section-1-introduction. Accessed November 11, 2018.

9. Campbell R. The five "rights" of clinical decision support. J AHIMA 2013;84:42–7.

10. Plebani M. Towards a new paradigm in laboratory medicine: the five rights. Clin Chem Lab Med 2016;54:1881–91.

11. Institute of Medicine (US) Committee on quality of health care in America. In: Kohn LT, Corrigan JM, Donaldson MS, editors. To err is human: building a safer health system. Washington, DC: National Academies Press (US); 2000.

12. Committee on Patient Safety and Health Information Technology, Institute of Medicine. Health IT and patient safety: building safer systems for better care. Washington, DC: National Academies Press (US); 2011.

13. Howard J, Clark EC, Friedman A, et al. Electronic health record impact on work burden in small, unaffiliated, community-based primary care practices. J Gen Intern Med 2013;28:107–13.

14. McAlearney AS, Robbins J, Hirsch A, et al. Perceived efficiency impacts following electronic health record implementation: an exploratory study of an urban community health center network. Int J Med Inform 2010;79:807–16.

15. West DR, James KA, Fernald DH, et al. Laboratory medicine handoff gaps experienced by primary care practices: a report from the shared networks of collaborative ambulatory practices and partners (SNOCAP). J Am Board Fam Med 2014;27:796–803.

16. Maillet É, Paré G, Currie LM, et al. Laboratory testing in primary care: a systematic review of health IT impacts. Int J Med Inform 2018;116:52–69.

17. Baron JM, Dighe AS. The role of informatics and decision support in utilization management. Clin Chim Acta 2014;427:196–201.

18. Hynes DM, Perrin RA, Rappaport S, et al. Informatics resources to support health care quality improvement in the Veterans Health Administration. J Am Med Inform Assoc 2004;11:344–50.

19. Henricks WH, Boyer PJ, Harrison JH, et al. Informatics training in pathology residency programs: proposed learning objectives and skill sets for the new millennium. Arch Pathol Lab Med 2003;127:1009–18.

20. Korpman RA. Using the computer to optimize human performance in health care delivery. Arch Pathol Lab Med 1987;111:637–45.

21. Weinstein RS, Bloom KJ. The pathologist as information specialist. Hum Pathol 1990;21:4–5.

22. Friedman BA. Informatics as a separate section within a department of pathology. Am J Clin Pathol 1990;94:S2–6.

23. Buffone GJ, Beck JR. Informatics: a subspecialty in pathology. Am J Clin Pathol 1993;100:75–81.

24. Becich MJ, Gross W, Schubert E, et al. Building an informatics training program for pathology. Semin Diagn Pathol 1994;11:237–44.

25. Elevitch FR. A pathologist is as a pathologist does: changing roles in a changing time. Arch Pathol Lab Med 1995;119:586–90.

26. Friedman BA. Pathology informatics ensuring a role as a "bit" player in laboratory medicine. Am J Clin Pathol 1996;105:S1–2.

27. Pelloso M, Basso D, Padoan A, et al. Computer-based-limited and personalised education management maximise appropriateness of vitamin D, vitamin B12 and folate retesting. J Clin Pathol 2016;69:777–83.
28. Rubinstein M, Hirsch R, Bandyopadhyay K, et al. Effectiveness of practices to support appropriate laboratory test utilization: a laboratory medicine best practices systematic review and meta-analysis. Am J Clin Pathol 2018;149:197–221.
29. Krintus M, Plebani M, Panteghini M. Improving clinical laboratory performance through quality indicators. Clin Biochem 2017;50:547–9.
30. Plebani M, Sciacovelli L, Aita A. Quality indicators for the total testing process. Clin Lab Med 2017;37:187–205.
31. Shahangian S, Snyder SR. Laboratory medicine quality indicators: a review of the literature. Am J Clin Pathol 2009;131:418–31.
32. Sciacovelli L, Sonntag O, Padoan A, et al. Monitoring quality indicators in laboratory medicine does not automatically result in quality improvement. Clin Chem Lab Med 2011;50:463–9.
33. Sciacovelli L, Aita A, Plebani M. Extra-analytical quality indicators and laboratory performances. Clin Biochem 2017;50:632–7.
34. Flegar-Meštrić Z, Perkov S, Radeljak A, et al. Risk analysis of the preanalytical process based on quality indicators data. Clin Chem Lab Med 2017;55:368–77.
35. Aita A, Sciacovelli L, Plebani M. Extra-analytical quality indicators - where to now? Clin Chem Lab Med 2018;57:127–33.
36. Kirchner MJ, Funes VA, Adzet CB, et al. Quality indicators and specifications for key processes in clinical laboratories: a preliminary experience. Clin Chem Lab Med 2007;45:672–7.
37. Ricós C, Biosca C, Ibarz M, et al. Quality indicators and specifications for strategic and support processes in laboratory medicine. Clin Chem Lab Med 2008;46:1189–94.
38. Llopis MA, Trujillo G, Llovet MI, et al. Quality indicators and specifications for key, analytical- extranalytical processes in the clinical laboratory. Five years' experience using the Six Sigma concept. Clin Chem Lab Med 2011;49:463–70.
39. Shcolnik W, de Oliveira CA, Sa de São Jose A, et al. Brazilian laboratory indicators program. Clin Chem Lab Med 2012;50:1923–34.
40. Badrick T, Gay S, Mackay M, et al. The key incident monitoring and management system - history and role in quality improvement. Clin Chem Lab Med 2018;56:264–72.
41. Sciacovelli L, Panteghini M, Lippi G, et al. Defining a roadmap for harmonizing quality indicators in Laboratory Medicine: a consensus statement on behalf of the IFCC Working Group "Laboratory Error and Patient Safety" and EFLM Task and Finish Group "Performance specifications for the extra-analytical phases". Clin Chem Lab Med 2017;55:1478–88.
42. Lippi G, Bonelli P, Rossi R, et al. Development of a preanalytical errors recording software. Biochem Med 2010;20:90–5.
43. Lippi G, Sciacovelli L, Simundic AM, et al. Innovative software for recording preanalytical errors in accord with the IFCC quality indicators. Clin Chem Lab Med 2017;55:e51–3.
44. Lundberg GD. When to panic over abnormal values. MLO Med Lab Obs 1972;4:47–54.
45. Piva E, Pelloso M, Penello L, et al. Laboratory critical values: automated notification supports effective clinical decision making. Clin Biochem 2014;47:1163–8.
46. Plebani M, Zaninotto M, Sciacovelli L, et al. Critical laboratory results: communication is just one of the problems. Am J Clin Pathol 2012;137:164.

47. Hawkins RC. Laboratory turnaround time. Clin Biochem Rev 2007;28:179–94.
48. Piva E, Sciacovelli L, Zaninotto M, et al. Evaluation of effectiveness of a computerized notification system for reporting critical values. Am J Clin Pathol 2009;131: 432–41.
49. Campbell CA, Horvath AR. Harmonization of critical result management in laboratory medicine. Clin Chim Acta 2014;432:135–47.
50. ISO. ISO 15189: Medical laboratories – particular requirements for quality and competence. Geneva (Switzerland): International Organization for Standardization (ISO); 2012.
51. Plebani M, Sciacovelli L, Bernardi D, et al. What information on measurement uncertainty should be communicated to clinicians, and how? Clin Biochem 2018;57: 18–22.
52. Plebani M. What information on quality specifications should be communicated to clinicians, and how? Clin Chim Acta 2004;346:25–35.
53. Fraser CG. Biological variation from principles to practice. Washington, DC: AACC Press; 2001.
54. JCGM 200:2012. International Vocabulary of Metrology – basic and general concepts and associated terms (VIM 3rd edition). Available at: www.bipm.org/en/publications/guides/. Accessed November 11, 2018.
55. Padoan A, Sciacovelli L, Aita A, et al. Measurement uncertainty in laboratory reports: a tool for improving the interpretation of test results. Clin Biochem 2018;57: 41–7.
56. Vasikaran S. Interpretative commenting. Clin Biochem Rev 2008;29:S99–103.
57. Gordon SC, Ping L. The assessment of interpretation of test results in laboratory medicine. Biochem Med 2009;19:146–53.
58. Buoro S, Da Rin G, Fanelli A, et al. Harmonization of interpretative comments in laboratory hematology reporting: the recommendations of Working Group on Diagnostic Hematology of the Italian Society of Clinical Chemistry and Clinical Molecular Biology (WGDH-SIBioC). Clin Chem Lab Med 2018. Available at: https://www.bipm.org/en/publications/guides/. Accessed November 11, 2018.
59. Lim EML, Sikaris KA, Gill J, et al. Quality assessment of interpretative commenting in clinical chemistry. Clin Chem 2004;50:632–7.
60. Koetsier S, Jones GRD, Badrick T. Safe reading of clinical pathology reports: the RCPAQAP Report Assessment Survey. Pathology 2016;48:357–62.
61. Tate JR, Johnson R, Barth J, et al. Harmonization of laboratory testing - current achievements and future strategies. Clin Chim Acta 2014;432:4–7.
62. Plebani M. Quality and future of clinical laboratories: the Vico's whole cyclical theory of the recurring cycles. Clin Chem Lab Med 2018;56:901–8.

Integrating Decision Support into a Laboratory Utilization Management Program

Kent Lewandrowski, MD

KEYWORDS

- Decision support • Utilization management • Clinical laboratory
- Utilization management tools

KEY POINTS

- Although laboratory testing typically accounts for only about 4% of total health care costs, the impact of laboratory testing on the downstream cost of care is pervasive.
- It has long been known that laboratory testing is overutilized, particularly the more common automated tests such as chemistry and hematology panels.
- Less commonly requested "esoteric" tests are usually much more expensive on a unit cost basis than routine panels, and therefore can add-up over time to a significant total cost.

INTRODUCTION

Health care expenditures in developed nations continue to rise, creating increasing pressure to improve efficiency and contain costs. Although laboratory testing typically accounts for only about 4% of total health care costs, the impact of laboratory testing on the downstream cost of care is pervasive. By some estimates, up to 70% of medical decisions are directly affected by laboratory test results.[1] It has long been known that laboratory testing is overutilized, particularly the more common automated tests, such as chemistry and hematology panels. For example, in a study in 1982 based on chart reviews, the authors reported that between 26.5% and 42.8% of tests were found to be unnecessary.[2] Less commonly requested "esoteric" tests are usually much more expensive on a unit cost basis than routine panels and therefore can add-up over time to a significant total cost. For example, at the Massachusetts General Hospital, we currently send out to reference laboratories about 7 million dollars per year in esoteric tests. The more recent and continuing introduction of very expensive genetic and molecular diagnostic tests, including large genetic panels

Disclosure: The author has nothing to disclose.
Department of Pathology, Massachusetts General Hospital, Gray 5, Fruit Street, Boston, MA 02114, USA
E-mail address: klewandrowski@partners.org

and whole-exome sequencing, has further added significant costs related to laboratory testing. This has led some third-party payers to restrict ordering of these tests or require cumbersome prior approvals before they will accept payment.

There are many reasons, other than reducing cost, why utilization management is important, as shown in **Box 1**. In the laboratory, unnecessary tests misdirect resources such as technologist labor and interfere with the processing of tests that are truly needed for patient care. Outside of the laboratory false-positive or -negative tests may result in undesirable clinical consequences, such as unnecessary work-ups or misdiagnoses. Given that many reference ranges for laboratory tests are often established as the normal population mean ±2 standard deviations, by statistical chance alone, 1 in 20 test results will fall outside of the normal range. This includes those tests that were unnecessary to begin with. Many clinicians find it difficult to ignore test results that are even slightly out of the normal range prompting further testing. Finally, from the patient's perspective, ordering of unnecessary tests contributes to iatrogenic anemia and may subject the patient to uncomfortable specimen collection procedures.

Physicians may order unnecessary tests for a variety of reasons, as shown in **Box 2**. In some cases the physician may not have up-to-date knowledge of the most appropriate test for a given clinical condition. For example, a physician might order a largely obsolete creatine kinase MB isoenzyme in a patient with chest pain in which troponin is the preferred test. Look-alike tests are also relatively common. An example would be 1,25-hydroxy (OH) vitamin D versus 25-OH vitamin D. The impact of defensive medicine on test utilization is well-known and pervasive, particularly in the United States. Most electronic order entry systems allow the physician to establish personal preference lists. Sometimes the wrong test is included in the preference list (eg, varicella zoster immunoglobulin M [IgM] versus IgG) or the preference list contains many tests, only some of which are relevant to any individual patient. In many hospitals, especially academic medical centers, test ordering patterns are established from historical trends or they may become embedded in the clinical "culture" of the service or organization. Inappropriate test-ordering habits are then passed down from one class of residents to the next. One example of this practice is the daily ordering by house staff of calcium/phosphate/magnesium on all patients on inpatient medical wards regardless of their clinical condition. Virtually all experienced physicians would consider this practice completely unnecessary. In some cases, test ordering is performed for the convenience of the physician. The practice of up-front ordering of daily laboratories is one example. Usually this takes the form of chemistry panels and a

---

Box 1
Reasons to control and manage laboratory utilization

1. Cost control
   On laboratory side:
   - Control operating budget
   - Alleviate labor shortages by reducing workload
   - Improve operations for needed testing
   Outside the laboratory
   - Reduce unnecessary work-ups, diagnostic studies, referrals, treatment delays, unnecessary treatments

2. Reduce diagnostic anemia

3. Ensure that patients get the correct test(s)

4. Reduce patient discomfort from unnecessary specimen collection procedures

---

Box 2

Examples of reasons why physicians order unnecessary laboratory tests

1. Lack of up-to-date knowledge of the most appropriate tests

2. Look-alike or sound-alike tests

3. Defensive medicine

4. Use of test preference lists including inclusion of inappropriate tests on preference lists

5. Adherence to historical or "cultural" test ordering practices

6. Convenience for physician

7. Concern of peer criticism for not ordering a test(s)

8. Pressure from patients to order certain tests

---

complete blood count ordered "daily until discontinued." In this way, the physician automates the ordering of laboratory tests such that they do not have to place orders on all their individual patients each day of hospitalization. Inexperienced physicians, particularly residents, may order laboratory tests of dubious necessity out of concern they might be criticized by their more senior peers during patient rounds. Finally, patients may pressure their physician to order certain tests. This situation is becoming common as more patients use the Internet to self-educate themselves about their (or their relatives) medical condition.

Most lay-persons believe that their physicians are generally competent and know what tests to order for a given clinical presentation. This is often not the case, especially when a physician is ordering tests for a condition outside of their specialty or expertise. Laposata and colleagues[3] reported a study on physician-ordering patterns in a special coagulation laboratory. The laboratory offers a variety of algorithms designed to select the correct tests and performs the appropriate sequence of tests for various special coagulation work-ups. Physicians who did not have access to the algorithms averaged 3.56 test ordering errors per patient requisition compared with 1.62 ordering errors for those who did have access to the algorithms. In another study by Miller and colleagues, a prospective review of genetic test orders by genetic counselors resulted in 26% of all test orders being changed from the original request.[4] Some laboratories have hired or contracted with genetic counselors to provide decision support for genetic tests.

Many strategies or "tools" have been described to assist in the implementation of utilization management initiatives, as described by Lewandrowski and colleagues[1] and in **Box 3**. Many of these rely on, or are facilitated by, clinical decision support. Clinical decision support can take many forms including requisition design (or electronic order entry field), performing automated reflex algorithms, establishing practice guidelines, implementing order entry "pop-ups," gatekeeping of selected tests, and providing an on-line laboratory handbook to name a few. The key to success is to choose the most appropriate strategy for any given utilization management initiative. An approach that works well for one type of initiative may prove a complete failure for a different type of initiative. In the discussion that follows, the role of decision support in many of these strategies will be discussed with specific examples. In many cases the laboratory will need access to a robust clinical informatics capability to acquire and analyze data and implement effective solutions. Ideally this capability would be in the form of a laboratory-based clinical pathologist who understands the medical aspects of laboratory testing and has advanced training in informatics.

Box 3
Utilization management tools to assist in implementation

Physician education and feedback
- Presentations at medical conferences
- Distributing literature on test guidelines
- Develop an electronic laboratory handbook with recommended laboratory work-ups
- Develop practice guidelines
- Identify and monitor "sound-alike" tests (eg, 25OH and 1,25OH vitamin D)
- Posting test costs or charges
- Retaining a laboratory-based genetic counselor
- Physician profiling and variation analysis
- Post "pending" tests to the electronic medical record

Restrictions on testing
- Discontinue obsolete tests (banning)
- Use of gatekeepers or prior authorization systems
- Restrict selected tests that can only be ordered by specific specialists
- Develop a list of tests that should never be ordered more than once (eg, genetic tests)
- Restrict inpatient send-out tests that are not relevant to the current hospitalization
- Capture and eliminate same-day duplicate tests
- Restrict the use of automatic orders for daily laboratory testing
- Establish a laboratory formulary

Requisition design

Validate and refine reference intervals to eliminate falsely abnormal tests

Develop admission templates

Order entry design
- Decision support
- Use of "pop-ups"

Develop algorithms and reflex testing protocols

Benchmarking against peer organizations

Clinical pathology consultative and interpretive services

Financial motivation including risk sharing and pay-for-performance

From Lewandrowski K, Baron J, Dighe A. Utilization management in the clinical laboratory: an introduction and overview. In: Lewandrowski K, editor. Utilization management in the clinical laboratory and other ancillary services. Cham (Switzerland): Springer; 2016. p. 17; with permission.

PHYSICIAN EDUCATION

Physician education has generally been viewed as a weak intervention, the effect of which is often short lived. This is particularly true when the education consists of a lecture or other educational material provided to a broad audience. In hospitals that have residency programs, the problem of providing physician education is compounded by the fact that there is a regular turnover of house staff as they complete their training. The key to determining whether physician education will be effective is to understand the reason for the inappropriate utilization, as shown in **Box 2**. For example, physician education would not be effective in reducing overutilization due to the practice of defensive medicine. On the other hand, if the problem is due to lack of knowledge on the part of the physician(s) or is the result of look-alike tests, then education may be a successful strategy. The next step is to determine the most appropriate form of education and whether it should be a one-time event or will require an ongoing intervention. At this stage it is important to understand who is ordering the test, why they are ordering it, and the test results. The problem may be limited to a single physician or specialty. If this were the case, the educational approach would be completely different than if the problem was widespread among several hundred or thousand physicians. For example, in our institution the preferred test for Babesiosis is examination of a thick and thin blood smear. In 2013, we observed that a significant number of serologic tests for Babesiosis were being sent out to our reference laboratory. A search of the ordering providers revealed that most of these tests were requested by a limited number of providers. The educational intervention was therefore directed at these physicians, which involved sending them a personalized e-mail describing the most optimal approach to testing for Babesiosis. We then set up a gatekeeping system in the laboratory to capture and redirect the occasional serologic tests requested by any of our other providers. The results of the intervention are shown in **Fig. 1**.

A key point concerning the success of educational interventions is that the educator must have credibility with the intended audience. In the case described above, we consulted with our division of infectious disease to get their support for the intervention. A second example of successful physician education involves ordering for vitamin D. In most cases 25OH vitamin D is the preferred test to assess vitamin D status. We noticed a seemingly large number of inpatient orders for 1,25OH vitamin D and began an investigation. This test was usually ordered by house staff without any concentration among any limited group of providers. There were 2 reasons why this test was being mistakenly ordered. First, it was a look-alike/sound-alike test. Second, medical students are taught that 1,25OH vitamin D is the most active vitamin and therefore is logically what one would order. In this case, we needed to educate a broad audience of physicians who also have a high rate of turnover. The decision support tool that we selected was an order entry "pop-up" as shown in **Fig. 2**. Pop-ups can be very effective if they are not overutilized because they provide decision support at the time that the physician is ready to place an order. However, excessive use of pop-ups will annoy physicians and lead to pop-up fatigue. Following implementation of the pop-up, 1,25OH vitamin D orders declined by 70% and remained low until we changed our hospital electronic medical record and implemented a new order entry system that did not include the pop-up message. Requests for 1,25OH vitamin D surged as shown in **Fig. 3**. The corrective action was to reinstate the pop-up alert

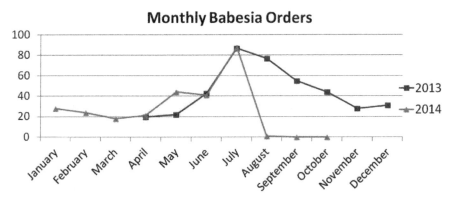

Fig. 1. Monthly Babesia serologies before (*line with boxes*) and after (*line with triangles*) educational/gatekeeping intervention.

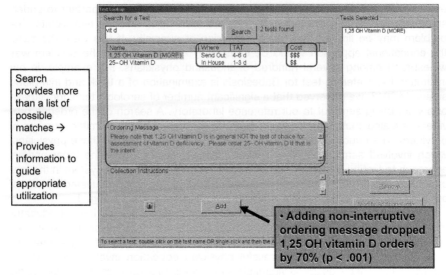

Fig. 2. Order entry screen display of a "pop-up" educational message when 1,25OH vitamin D is ordered by a clinician.

and the test requests declined accordingly. This initiative illustrates several key decision support caveats:

1. Some educational initiatives must be maintained to provide continuous feedback to the providers especially among physicians with a high turnover rate.
2. Trend anomaly monitoring is important as changes occurring within an organization can recreate misutilization that had previously been resolved.
3. Decision support cannot only reduce overutilization, but it can also ensure that the patient gets the correct test, in this case 25OH vitamin D.

Notice also in **Fig. 2** that there is a display of the relative cost of the 2 tests displayed in dollar signs ($$ and $$$). Physicians are often unaware of the cost of laboratory tests.

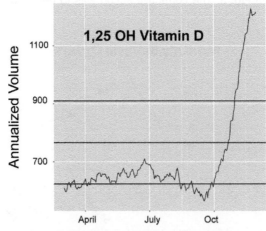

Fig. 3. Monthly orders for 1,25OH vitamin D on inpatients following changeover to a new order entry system without an educational "pop-up."

Posting costs (or alternatively charges) has been shown to have a modest but significant affect on test utilization.[5] It is important to understand the difference between cost and charges. The cost to perform a laboratory test including labor, reagents, and consumables is usually much less than the charge for the test. Laboratory charges are usually set to maximize reimbursement and may bear little relationship to actual costs.

ON-LINE LABORATORY HANDBOOK

Many laboratories have developed an on-line electronic laboratory handbook that includes information such as the test menu, specimen requirements, turnaround times, and normal reference values. However, once physicians become accustomed to using the handbook it can then be leveraged as a tool for decision support. **Fig. 4** shows a screen shot from our laboratory handbook, which appears when the test anti-endomysial antibody, an expensive send-out test, is selected. An ordering message seems to encourage the physician to order tissue transglutaminase instead. Note also (arrow) the handbook contains a link to our reference laboratory that includes additional interpretation of the anti-endomysial antibody test if the clinician chooses to proceed with the order.

PRACTICE GUIDELINES

Practice guidelines are becoming increasingly important to assist physicians in evidence-based medicine. Practice guidelines may be developed by many different organizations including the government, professional organizations, and those that are developed locally within an individual organization. The keys to successful practice guidelines are that they must be authoritative, widely disseminated, readily available at the time of the clinical encounter, and convenient to implement. Practice guidelines should help physicians manage clinical problems and make it easier for clinicians to do the right thing and discourage wasteful practices. There are many ways that practice guidelines can be made available in a convenient format for physicians. In the simplest case the clinical laboratory can implement reflex algorithms, whereby the clinician can request the algorithm rather than ordering all possible tests that might be required individually. Typically, this eliminates tests that become unnecessary based on the results of initial testing and guides the laboratory work-up to a logical conclusion. For example, **Fig. 5** shows the Massachusetts General Hospital algorithm

Endomysial IgA antibody		MGH Order Code: MAENDM
Site	MGH	
System	SUNQUEST LAB	
Epic Lab Code	LAB774	
Local Code	MAENDM	
Specimen	BLOOD	
Container	Gold top tube, plain, gel, 5 ml	
Turnaround Time	1–3 d	
Order Message	NOTE: For initial screening of celiac disease please do not order Endomysial IgA but instead order Tissue Transglutaminase IgA. It is currently recommended in most screening algorithms for celiac disease.	
Test Usage	Endomysial autoantibodies are highly specific for gluten-sensitive enteropathies such as celiac disease and dermatitis herpetiformis. It reacts with tissue transglutaminase.	
Additional Information	Additional information from reference laboratory	

Fig. 4. Screen shot of on-line laboratory handbook when anti-endomysial antibody test is requested. The "order message" provides educational guidance for the clinician.

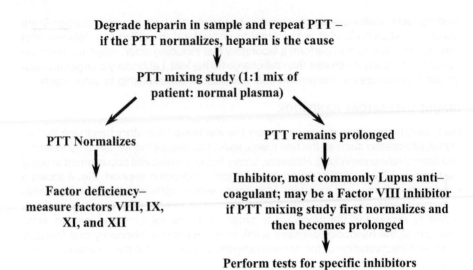

**Degrade heparin in sample and repeat PTT –
if the PTT normalizes, heparin is the cause**

**PTT mixing study (1:1 mix of
patient: normal plasma)**

PTT Normalizes

**Factor deficiency–
measure factors VIII, IX,
XI, and XII**

PTT remains prolonged

**Inhibitor, most commonly Lupus anti–
coagulant; may be a Factor VIII inhibitor
if PTT mixing study first normalizes and
then becomes prolonged**

**Perform tests for specific inhibitors
suggested by results of PTT mixing study**

Fig. 5. Reflex algorithm for the evaluation of a prolonged partial thromboplastin time (PTT).

for the evaluation of a prolonged partial thromboplastin time (PTT). Rather than ordering all possible tests up-front, the physician simply orders "prolonged PTT evaluation" and the laboratory automatically performs the evaluation while sequentially eliminating unnecessary tests.

Our institution has implemented many on-line decision support practice guidelines to aid in clinical decision making. One of these is our Primary Care Office Insight Web site that contains many practice guidelines across different areas of clinical specialties, as shown in **Fig. 6**. The Web site is readily available at the click of the mouse on any hospital workstation. Many professional organizations have published on-line practice guidelines. An example of one of these is the Infectious Disease Society of America guidelines available at http://www.idsociety.org/PracticeGuidelines/. Decision support can facilitate making professional organization guidelines readily available such that local physicians can access them easily and conveniently at the time of the clinical encounter.

REQUISITION (OR ORDER ENTRY FIELD) DESIGN

The way tests are displayed on a test requisition or order entry field can have a significant impact on test ordering by physicians. Our previous order entry system had a "quick pick" screen that displayed all commonly ordered tests to make routine orders convenient for our physicians. To select the desired tests they simply checked the boxes next to the test name. One test, lactate dehydrogenase, was included on the quick pick screen. Although this test has some specific indications it was being significantly overutilized by our house staff physicians. Removing the test from the quick pick screen resulted in a dramatic decrease in orders for this test as shown in **Fig. 7**.

PHYSICIAN PROFILING

Physician profiling and analysis of practice variation can be used as a form of education/decision support if it provides useful feedback to allow individual physicians to

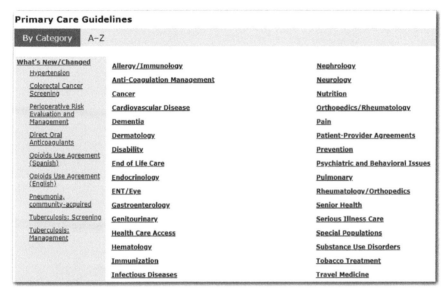

Fig. 6. Partners Healthcare Primary Care Office Insight (PCOI) practice guidelines screenshot.

modify their laboratory testing practices. Many studies have documented wide variations in physician practices that could not be explained by differences in acuity or the case mix of the patient populations.[6,7] Obtaining reliable physician profiling data usually requires a robust informatics capability that is able to distinguish true practice variation from differences in patient volume, patient case mix, and other factors. As part of a utilization effort targeting testing for tick-borne illnesses, we analyzed which physicians were ordering serologic testing for *Anaplasma/Ehrlichia*, a test we were trying to discourage in favor of polymerase chain reaction-based testing. **Fig. 8** shows the utilization of the serologic test by the most frequent user (Dr. X) before (2015) and after (2016) showing the provider their profile versus other comparable physicians.

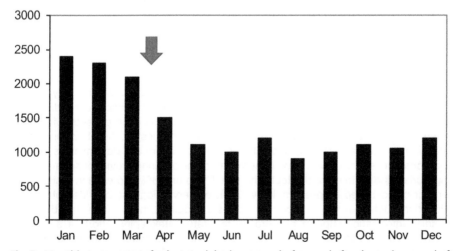

Fig. 7. Monthly test requests for lactate dehydrogenase before and after (*arrow*) removal of the test from a "quick pick" screen.

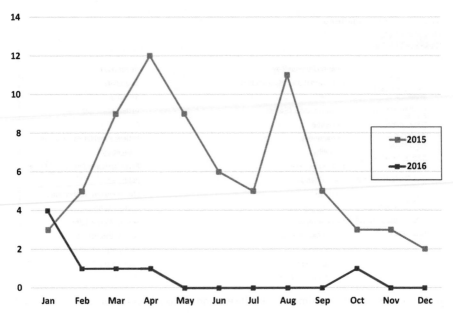

Fig. 8. Impact of physician profiling. Monthly orders by a single clinician for *Anaplasma/Ehrlichia* serologies before (2015) and after (2016) physician profiling.

GATEKEEPING

Gatekeeping is another decision support tool that may be used to decrease overutilization and enhance physician education. Tests that are most amenable to gatekeeping have the following characteristics:

1. The test has established indications but is overutilized.
2. The test is expensive and is not high volume: gatekeeping requires time for the laboratory director to intervene in test ordering 1 test at a time. The savings from not doing the test should exceed the cost of the gatekeeping event. High volume tests are not suitable to gatekeeping as the time required to intervene in multiple tests per day is prohibitive.
3. Misuse of the test results from physicians misunderstanding the appropriate indications for the test and its potential alternatives.

As one example of gatekeeping we identified blood-based quantitative polymerase chain reaction testing for herpes simplex virus as a test that had clear indications (mainly pediatrics) but was being overutilized, especially in adult patients. Most test orders were from adult patients. Each time a test was requested, the laboratory director would review the history in the electronic medical record and determine its level of appropriateness. The director would then contact the ordering provider and review the appropriate indications for the test. The result was an 88% decrease in tests being sent for blood-based herpes simplex virus. The intervention also provided physician education such that the number of requests requiring intervention has declined steadily. Informatics support can greatly facilitate gatekeeping efforts if a system can be developed that can gather data from multiple sources such as the laboratory information system and the electronic medical record. The gatekeeper can therefore be provided with most if not all of the required information up-front to determine if an intervention is warranted. For example, there are some tests that we automatically approve on immunosuppressed patients whereas requests on immunocompetent patients triggers an intervention. The gatekeeper needs to know the patient, the provider, and the hospital unit from which the test originated (most immunosuppressed patients are located on a limited number of inpatient units). If the test originated from one of these inpatient units, the gatekeeper approves the test without an intervention thus avoiding wasting time on interventions of low yield.

CLINICAL LABORATORY CONSULTATIONS

Consultations performed by laboratory directors provide another source of decision support and allow direct physician education. These can take many forms, from so-called curbside consults in person or over the phone, written consults by e-mail, and formal written consults that become part of the electronic medical record as part of a laboratory medicine interpretive service. In a survey of physicians who used a laboratory medicine consult service, Laposata and colleagues reported the following responses[3]:

1. 80% of physicians stated the consultation saved time and improved the diagnostic process.
2. 59% stated the interpretation reduced the time to diagnosis.
3. 72% stated the interpretation reduced the number of laboratory tests.
4. 72% stated the interpretation helped to prevent a misdiagnosis.

Many laboratory-based consultations are also billable as a professional service, which helps to offset the cost of the service. An example of a laboratory interpretation from our institution is shown in **Box 4**.

DEFINING OVERUTILIZATION

One ongoing challenge regarding utilization management is determining what inappropriate utilization actually is. As described by Lewandrowski and colleagues,[1] "In many cases there is no consensus on what testing is, or is not, appropriate." Although clinical guidelines exist for some types of testing, often there is no peer-reviewed literature defining appropriate test utilization. For example, how often

---

Box 4
Example of a clinical laboratory coagulation interpretation

Patient
    54-year-old woman with deep vein thrombosis undergoing a hypercoagulation work-up

Interpretation
    A low value was obtained for functional and free protein S. It is known that factor VIII levels in excess of 200% will artifactually depress the functional protein S value. For that reason, a factor VIII activity was performed and found to be elevated by more than 200%. Fibrinogen, factor VIII and C4b-binding protein are elevated during acute phase reactions. It is likely that C4b-binding protein is elevated in the present study. Elevations in C4b-binding protein decrease the free protein S. The protein S assays should be repeated when the patient has recovered from the acute phase reaction, at a time when the patient has not received Coumadin for at least 10 days and has not received estrogen therapy for at least 2 months

Interpretation impact: prevents falsely low protein S value from triggering further work-up. Provides advice on repeat testing.

should a typical patient hospitalized with community-acquired pneumonia have a complete blood count test. Walraven performed a systematic literature review of studies that provided and applied criteria for inappropriate utilization. They concluded that many studies used implicit or explicit criteria that did not meet acceptable methodological standards.[8-10] In a follow-on study by Hauser, the authors commented that in the past many studies used subjective or locally defined definitions of appropriate. However, literature consensus of what is appropriate has improved, and advances in database technologies, as opposed to chart reviews, have facilitated utilization audits.[8] In our experience, determining what is inappropriate utilization is often impossible or, when there are data, they are often inconclusive. In most cases we rely on local clinical experts to provide guidance or meet with clinicians to try to reach a consensus. Invariably this process is based more on intuition and experience rather than true evidence, but we have nonetheless have had a number of successes. Lacking clear evidence-based guidelines, some patterns of testing may develop locally and become ingrained in the culture of the organization. For example, house staff in many academic medical centers have developed informal "guidelines" for daily laboratory tests, or so-called "daily labs" on inpatients. Usually these include a complete blood count, a basic metabolic panel, and calcium/phosphate/magnesium testing. Most experienced physicians would agree that the required laboratory tests for a given patient should be assessed on an ongoing basis and be individualized to the needs of the patient. In a review of test ordering patterns in our institution we observed a large number of orders for routine laboratory tests as "daily until discontinued" particularly on the inpatient medicine service. To address this problem, we formed an interdisciplinary ad hoc committee with membership from pathology and internal medicine. The team developed a guideline for when daily laboratory testing was appropriate (eg, patient on warfarin or heparin). Our guideline was not based on hard evidence but rather was developed by forming a consensus among experienced senior physicians. The guideline was approved by the hospital Medical Policy Committee. We then set up an order entry pop-up to display the guideline and ask for the reason when daily laboratory testing was requested. We then set up a computerized audit by individual provider. Any provider who ordered 4 or more non-guideline-compliant daily orders in a prior week was sent a personal e-mail describing the guideline and noting its approval by the Medical Policy Committee. Over a 33-month period, annualized daily order requests declined from 25,000 to 10,000.[11]

SUMMARY

Utilization management is increasingly important to control health care costs and to ensure that patients receive the most appropriate tests. Most utilization management initiatives either require, or are facilitated by, clinical decision support. To be successful, utilization management programs must be supported by a robust clinical informatics capability. Ideally, this will be led by a laboratory-based physician who understands the clinical aspects of laboratory testing and has advanced training in informatics.

REFERENCES

1. Lewandrowski K, Baron J, Dighe A. Utilization management in the clinical laboratory: an introduction and overview. In: Lewandrowski K, editor. Utilization management in the clinical laboratory and other ancillary services. Cham (Switzerland): Springer; 2016. p. 7–29.

2. McConnell T, Berger P, Dayton H, et al. Professional review of laboratory utilization. Hum Pathol 1982;13:399–403.
3. Laposata ME, Laposata M, Van Cott EM, et al. Physician survey of a laboratory medicine interpretive service and evaluation of the influence of interpretations on laboratory test ordering. Arch Pathol Lab Med 2004;128:1424–7.
4. Miller C, Krautscheid P, Baldwin E, et al. Genetic counselor review of genetic test orders in a reference laboratory reduces unnecessary testing. Am J Med Genet A 2014;164:1094–100.
5. Feldman L, Shihab H, Thiemann D, et al. Impact of providing fee data on laboratory test ordering. JAMA Intern Med 2013;173:903–8.
6. Welsh G, Miller M, Welch P. Physician profiling: an analysis of inpatient practice patterns in Florida and Oregon. N Engl J Med 1994;330:607–12.
7. Wennberg J, Gittelson A. Small area variations in health care delivery. Science 1973;182:1102–8.
8. Walraven C, Naylor D. Do we know what inappropriate laboratory utilization is: a systematic review of laboratory clinical audits. JAMA 1998;280:550–8.
9. Hauser R, Shirts B. Do we know what inappropriate laboratory utilization is: an expanded systematic review of laboratory clinical audits. Am J Clin Pathol 2014;141:774–83.
10. Grumet G. Health care rationing through inconvenience. N Engl J Med 1989;321:607–11.
11. Rudolf JW, Dighe AS, Coley CM, et al. Analysis of daily laboratory orders at a large urban academic center: a multifaceted approach to changing test ordering patterns. Am J Clin Pathol 2017;148:128–35.

Decision Support to Enhance Automated Laboratory Testing by Leveraging Analytical Capabilities

J. Mark Tuthill, MD

KEYWORDS

- Business analytics • Clinical decision support • Laboratory automation
- Dashboards • Artificial intelligence • Learning health systems

KEY POINTS

- Understand data science and the four types of data analytics.
- Recognize that laboratory clinical decision support leverages several types of data analytics to support business processes.
- Describe the practical tools that support laboratory clinical decision support, such as real-time dashboards, autovalidation, and reflex testing.
- Visualize future possibilities for clinical decision support leveraging new developments in artificial intelligence leading to learning systems.

INTRODUCTION

Business analytics, clinical decision support, machine learning, artificial intelligence. How do these buzz words impact running a modern laboratory? The answer is, profoundly. Without analytical capabilities, a laboratory is effectively deaf, dumb, and blind. It is through the use of data analytics that the modern laboratory is most effectively and efficiently managed. This includes impact on daily operations and laboratory performance, and more sophisticated opportunities to predict in advance not only health system business needs and laboratory performance requirements, but new opportunities to impact patient care in novel ways. As computational power continues to increase, and software is developed to analyze and synthesize data into information, knowledge is created, and ultimately a higher order of information, wisdom. Although this may be hyperbole to a degree, what is clear is that laboratories that leverage the data they create on a daily basis to change the way they work and support clinical

Disclosure: The author has nothing to disclose.
Henry Ford Health System, 2799 W. Grand Boulevard, K-6 Pathology, Detroit, MI 48202, USA
E-mail address: Mtuthil1@hfhs.org

Clin Lab Med 39 (2019) 259–267
https://doi.org/10.1016/j.cll.2019.01.005
0272-2712/19/© 2019 Elsevier Inc. All rights reserved.

practitioners are more efficient, successful, and more deeply valued by hospital leadership.

Henry Ford Health System (HFHS) Pathology and Laboratory Medicine (PALM) has long used data generated from routine testing to support not only decisions about laboratory operations but to communicate to clinical departments the value and impact of laboratory testing on their patient services. Because hospitals are tightly connected departmental ecosystems, it is well recognized that laboratory testing is key to effective patient care. Whether the impact of turnaround time (TAT) on emergency room throughput or infectious disease reporting to monitor nosocomial infection rates, nearly all modern laboratories provide analytical information that impacts patient care. In fact, some of this reporting is required by government and regulatory agencies. Good examples of this are requirements for reporting cancer; infectious disease rates for certain organisms; and analytes, such as lead levels.

These primary analytical reporting requirements have continued to grow over time and can consume a significant amount of time and effort by laboratories, but are actually a limited starting point compared with future opportunities. Imagine, rather than reacting to nosocomial infection outbreaks after the fact, that analytics could predict such outbreaks proactively or least provide real-time alerts to an increasing trend. Further imagine that panels of laboratory tests could be analyzed using artificial intelligence algorithms to predict other values that were not directly tested. It is beginning to be seen that such algorithms are not only plausible, but possible and clinically effective.[1] Such algorithms save time and money by eliminating expensive reference laboratory testing.

The application of laboratory data analytics will be far reaching as more sophisticated tools become available and easier to use. Some of these tools allow integration of data from disparate systems to be leveraged in unique ways. Rather than just looking at daily laboratory operations, such analytical paradigms allow for laboratory data to be used to look at provider utilization and performance, patient outcomes, care modeling, and financial forecasting to mention a few. This is the next generation of laboratory analytics.

This article addresses the historical, current, and future state of laboratory analytics using examples, and offering a framework to organize thinking around analytical capabilities. This helps the reader understand where they are in the continuum of data analysis, suggesting steps toward the future.

UNDERSTANDING AND ORGANIZING ANALYTICS CONCEPTS: DATA SCIENCE

Business analytics or data analytics has become increasingly formalized. This has resulted in professionals with specialization in data science at the undergraduate and post-graduate level.[2] As this field develops, the lexicon of data analytics has become more formalized using recognized nomenclature that should be understood by laboratorians specifically and health care professionals in general. The primary driver for the growth of data science has been the increase in computing power and data storage, and the development of sophisticated vendor solutions and open source technology. This includes leveraging cloud-based solutions, Internet technology, robust databases, and data warehouses. This technology, in conjunction with increasing pressure on laboratories to address costs and efficiency in the current regulatory environment, has created a desire for laboratories to better understand their work, and to improve their workflow. Whereas clinical decision support (CDS) in the clinical arena typically focuses on efficacious use of laboratory services by health care practitioners, within the laboratory such support systems are directed at preanalytical, analytical, and postanalytical aspects of diagnostic testing.

Data science has recognized four basic types of analytics[3]
- Descriptive analytics: What happened?
- Diagnostic analytics: Why it happened?
- Predictive analytics: What will happen?
- Prescriptive analytics: How can we make it happen?

Each of these types of analytics has increasing sophistication in technical requirements and impact. Higher order analytics will lead to the deployment of applications that leverage artificial intelligence and machine learning culminating in "learning systems" that are the outcome of effectively deployed prescriptive analytics. To date most laboratory CDS is driven by descriptive analytics in combination with diagnostic analytics, but predictive and prescriptive analytics are beginning to be developed.

CLINICAL DECISION SUPPORT IN THE AUTOMATED LABORATORY: OPERATIONAL IMPACTS

Leveraging data analytics in the laboratory provides the tools that support operations and best practices (**Table 1**). This is different than how one views CDS in the clinical arena. Looking at such basic data, such as laboratory testing, TAT can provide an end-to-end example. When one looks at TAT at the level of descriptive analytics, one uses the raw data in combination with expected best practices to determine whether the desired outcome was met. That is, what happened? If the desired TAT metric was not achieved, diagnostic analytics are used to determine why the goal failed to be achieved. For example, preanalytical factors, such as sample integrity (eg, hemolysis or a clotted sample) or transport time, can be identified. Using predictive analytics, one may model how changes can improve the process. Finally, in a finely tuned system leveraging artificial intelligence and machine learning such an analytical system could suggest the answer. For example, a recommendation to add a new courier route at a given time of day. Perhaps even automatically identifying a practitioner with a higher number of preanalytical defects allowing just in time education to be provided that is directly related to the type of defect experienced.

In the preceding simple example, the operational requirement is to capture the appropriate data elements that can be processed by a pipeline leading from raw description to sophisticated responses and interventions, that is, prescription. To date this has been challenging for laboratories. Although most laboratories leverage descriptive analytics in their CDS processes, the data leveraged are typically static and historic. That is, one is assessing and reacting to yesterday's information today. With such design approaches one can leverage diagnostic analytics to demonstrate

Table 1		
CDS systems in the laboratory and the data analytical type		
CDS System	**Data Type**	**Analytical Type**
TAT dashboard	Static	Descriptive
TAT dashboard	Dynamic	Descriptive, diagnostic
Volume dashboard	Static	Descriptive
Volume dashboard	Dynamic	Descriptive, diagnostic, predictive, prescriptive
Critical value call back	Static or dynamic	Descriptive, diagnostic
Reflex testing	Dynamic	Descriptive, diagnostic, prescriptive
Autoverification	Dynamic	Descriptive, diagnostic, predictive, prescriptive
Learning systems	Dynamic	Descriptive, diagnostic, predictive, prescriptive

a transport delay or clotted specimen, and may even be able to model how changes to the system could be implemented, but there is little hope of a dynamic, prescriptive intervention, never mind a learning system. For this to occur, data from the automated laboratory must be continuously analyzed in conjunction with information from other systems such as inbound clinical orders, data from the LIS (Laboratory Information System), instruments, and even the automation line control software. As a result of the reliance on static, historic data, few laboratories have achieved an end-to-end analytics pipeline. However, as practitioners become more mature and sophisticated in applying data analytics, the beginnings of such a pipeline are able to be conceptualized. A key constraint to this work is not only the ability to capture the required data points, but also the human resources to focus on these efforts.

REFLEX TESTING AND TESTING CASCADES

Although the TAT example presented is a common day-to-day CDS monitor, one can imagine more sophisticated applications of CDS within and outside the laboratory. These include such behaviors as reflex testing, leading to testing cascades where the results of one test may lead automatically to the performance of another.[4] The classic example is the reflex ordering of a ferritin in the case of microcytic anemia to rule in iron deficiency. In the automated core laboratory, this may result in a sample being automatically retrieved from a storage stockyard for additional testing, versus the manual approach. This is a real, albeit simple, example of laboratory CDS. Leveraging the concepts of data science, it is not difficult to imagine more sophisticated examples, such as alerting a clinician that the antibiotic resistance of a bacterial isolate is not congruent with a patient's current medication. A learning system may even suggest the most appropriate therapy for a given patient taking into account multiple variables, such as kidney function, allergy status, and the patient's problem list.

One can imagine many such scenarios, but most still fall into descriptive and diagnostic analytics, with predictive analytics and modeling being carried out offline by a human. As more data are gathered from different areas of the patient care environment, analyzed and learned from, the game will change. Imagine, for example, that the correct initial antibiotic could be predicted based on multiple historical data points with a statistical degree of confidence. Although this is the purpose for publishing the antibiotic resistance profile for organism in an environment, such information is descriptive or a best diagnostic. Only when multiple factors are taken into account can such models become increasingly predictive and prescriptive.

THE USE OF ANALYTICS AND CLINICAL DECISION SUPPORT BY HENRY FORD HEALTH SYSTEM PATHOLOGY AND LABORATORY MEDICINE
Static Data and Dashboards

Historically, PALM has long used data to help make clinical decisions around laboratory testing, defect elimination, and process improvement. Leveraging static TAT and defect reports the laboratory has been able to work with clinical customers to support their needs. One early example was monitoring TAT for markers of cardiac damage for samples coming from the emergency room; previously creatine kinase-myocardial band, and currently cardiac troponin. It is well recognized that TAT of these tests directly impacts emergency room wait time and throughput.[5] TAT metrics were typically produced as daily reports showing the prior day's success or failure in meeting a TAT threshold for a given analyte. These reports were produced by extracting the prior day's laboratory data and descriptively analyzing them for the outcome: pass or fail. If there was a failure to meet the desired TAT threshold, additional data could be analyzed to determine the reason for failure. Often times this required additional information to be generated or queries into other systems. Because these data were static and a day old, no direct intervention was possible at the time of failure. More recently this information is presented on more refined paper dashboards distributed by email, but effectively it is still historical and static.

Autoverification

The use of autoverification or autovalidation is one of the earliest and most impactful applications of CDS in the clinical laboratory. It is not well recognized by most outside the laboratory what is required to release results downstream. Basic result reporting requirements, such as valid quality assurance for a given testing run and the relationship of test results to a reference range, have long required manual intervention to review test results to determine the suitability of releasing them. Autoverification mitigates this effort by allowing rules to be established for the automatic release of results.[6] For example, if a result is within the normal range, and the quality assurance was valid, the result can be released directly. This is a powerful form of laboratory CDS that significantly impacts laboratory resources and improves TAT. Imagine having to review thousands of normal test results before releasing them. The autoverification process is based on descriptive analytical algorithms and is simple to implement because most LIS have this functionality built-in. Autoverification has direct impact on the resources required for testing. By removing "normal results" from the review stream, laboratory personnel are better able to focus on important, abnormal, and impactful values. Autoverification rules can be quite sophisticated going beyond quality assurance to include delta checks, completion of reflex testing, and results of additional testing that may be a required part of a testing cascade. Not only does this eliminate errors of omission, but it ensures that clinicians get fully completed information at the time results release, eliminating iterative review of the medical record.

Critical Values

Laboratory testing that results in values that are of high clinical impact for patient care are one of the most disruptive, challenging aspects of providing laboratory services. So called "critical values" not only are important for quality patient care, but also have significant requirements from regulatory bodies impacting laboratory accreditation, and justly so. The failure to report a critical result to a provider in a timely fashion can negatively impact patient care.[7,8] Examples of this abound. Systems that support a closed loop communication process between laboratory and clinicians have been difficult to implement. The process actually requires significant CDS. From the identification of a critical value, to validation of the result, identification of a provider, contacting the provider, communicating the details for the result and its critical nature, documenting the callback, and significant rework for any step in the process, the process can take hours (**Box 1**). If one were to follow the paradigms of data analytics, one might see the problem in a completely different light.

Recognizing the critical value is a descriptive analytical process; the callback process, diagnostic analytics; and leaping to the prescriptive aspects of the process, and the business intelligence required for the intercommunications, it is no wonder the problem has been so difficult to solve. If such results could be anticipated earlier in the testing cycle the volume of calls might drop using predicative analytics to adjust rules for particular patient populations, and yet identify truly emergent results.

Recently, process improvements at HFHS PALM have led to significant reworking of the callback process. We discovered key aspects of this process are highly amenable to CDS. For example, the volume of testing is directly related to critical value

---

Box 1
Steps in the critical value call back process

1. Identify a critical value
2. Validate the truth of the result
3. Identify the provider to contact
4. Contact the provider
5. Document the communication with read back by the provider
6. Iteratively rework failed steps

---

generation. Therefore, volume dashboards can be leveraged to anticipate staffing and the complexity of communication. Using descriptive diagnostics, we can recognize the reasons we have critical values and the details around their origins. Predicting and modeling support requirements led us to new efficiencies with prescriptive knowledge leading to better patient outcomes and more efficient provider communication.

Dynamic Dashboards and Expanded Data Feeds

More recently, HFHS PALM has begun to develop dynamic data feeds to an analytical pipeline that is continuously updated. This allows for deviations in the preanalytical or analytical processes to be recognized in near real time allowing for more rapid intervention. Although these dashboards need to be monitored, they can be viewed on screen, with dynamic refreshing. Furthermore, without any additional query, the details behind a summary dashboard can be drilled into to get to the details. As designed, the details can include additional data elements that are helpful at the level of diagnostic analytics. This includes data from third-party systems that not only aid understanding as to why a deviation occurred, but may aid in its resolution. Although we are still short of predictive or prescriptive models, dynamic data feeding our pipeline is the first step.

Yet another example related to the TAT is our use of ePending logs or TAT outlier monitor dashboards. This information is displayed dynamically on large screens that effectively function as electronic Andon boards. When a given analyte from a location exceeds its threshold, it can be visually highlighted on the TAT outlier monitor indicating a problem. Because this is the same pipeline providing the overall TAT report the data can be drilled into to visualize and diagnose the reason for the threshold failure. These TAT outlier monitor dashboards now include detailed information coming from the automation line, such as current sample location or testing that shares tubes. This aids in resolving deviations in real time.

Dynamic Volume Reports

However, the real value of the dynamic data pipeline derives from the ability to view data continuously and over time (currently 1 month). This allows one to relate laboratory performance dynamically and across time without the need to generate new queries to the LIS. This also allows us to look at the data iteratively using filters and refinements within the pipeline. The ability to visualize trends begins to allow predictive analytics as a CDS tool in the laboratory. Even a simple dashboard, such as volume of orders by location, for current versus historic orders is profound, facilitating improved allocation of resources, shift planning, reagent ordering, and so forth. For example, if one notes a current high volume of orders from a given site compared with its historic normal, the laboratory can react prospectively to support service requirements.

UTILIZATION

Laboratory test utilization is another example where moving from purely descriptive to prescriptive analytics has an impact on the efficient use of laboratory services allowing for better CDS. Many of the articles in this issue describe the impact of CDS tools, such alerts and ordering cascades or best practices to appropriately direct use of laboratory services. Detailed, real-time analysis of utilization can help to identify interventions that could be considered for future CDS activities. For example, capturing and storing laboratory test orders, results, patient demographics, and International Classification of Diseases information not only allows the laboratory to monitor services, but can also provide alerts and summary information. An example of this is monitoring testing that can directly impact patients. For example, monitoring the lack of hemoglobin A_{1c} testing (HbA_{1c}) in a patient with an International Classification of Diseases code of diabetes for a given calendar year. When this is taken to the level of prescriptive analytics such a system would alert the clinician, or perhaps even the patient, that important laboratory testing has not been done. And this is just the beginning. Perhaps the lack of HbA_{1c} testing could be determined to be a surrogate marker for other aspects of missing patient care. Thus, a missing HbA_{1c} is predictive, and potentially prescriptive for other forms of intervention. Perhaps this is not a medical problem but a social one, such as a patient having lost insurance, or being unable to afford medication, thus the lack of HbA_{1c} is predictive of a health care delivery problem, not just a missing test. As another example, imagine the power of monitoring the care events that follow a positive pregnancy test, particularly if the patient never comes back. In fact, such systematic intervention and data analytics to the level of prescriptive analytics are the unpinning of what has become to be referred as "Lab 2.0."[9]

FUTURE VISION: LEARNING HEALTH SYSTEMS

Taken in toto, an analytics pipeline that goes beyond descriptive and diagnostic analytics and begins to leverage predictive and prescriptive combined with machine learning and artificial intelligence achieves a new level of sophistication: a learning system. A learning health system is defined by the Institute of Medicine as one in which: "science, informatics, incentives, and culture are aligned for continuous improvement and innovation, with best practices seamlessly embedded in the delivery process and new knowledge captured as an integral by-product of the delivery experience."[10–12] The process cycle of such systems has been described as including the following steps:

- Assemble
- Analyze
- Interpret
- Feedback
- Change

CDS as viewed through the prism of a learning system leads to a vision of a spontaneous, dynamic environment for modeling and implementing CDS that may have been otherwise unappreciated. Could such systems someday provide for sophisticated CDS that exceed the limits of human observation?

SUMMARY

CDS in the laboratory derives from the data analytical process model. Such analyses, although dependent on descriptive and diagnostic analytics, will ultimately leverage more sophisticated analytics including predictive and prescriptive analytics. The culmination of the effective implementation of such systems will lead to the development of learning health systems within the clinical laboratory. Leveraging this information is essential to the efficient operation of an automated core laboratory. Examples of CDS in the laboratory have been discussed in the context of data analytics models that allow the reader to organize the implementation of such processes and CDS tools.

REFERENCES

1. Colón-Franco JM, Bossuyt PMM, Algeciras-Schimnich A, et al. Current and emerging multianalyte assays with algorithmic analyses: are laboratories ready for clinical adoption? Clin Chem 2018;64(6):885–91. Available at: http://clinchem.aaccjnls.org/content/64/6/885.
2. National Academies of Sciences, Engineering, and Medicine, Division of Behavioral and Social Sciences and Education, Board on Science Education, Division on Engineering and Physical Sciences, Committee on Applied and Theoretical Statistics, Board on Mathematical Sciences and Analytics, Computer Science and Telecommunications Board, Committee on Envisioning the Data Science Discipline: The Undergraduate Perspective. Washington, DC: National Academies Press (US); 2018. Available at: https://www.ncbi.nlm.nih.gov/pubmed/30407778.
3. Khalifa M. Health analytics types, functions and levels: a review of literature. Stud Health Technol Inform 2018;251:137–40. Available at: https://www.ncbi.nlm.nih.gov/pubmed/29968621.
4. Ferraro S, Panteghini M. The role of laboratory in ensuring appropriate test requests. Clin Biochem 2017;50(10–11):555–61. Available at: https://www.ncbi.nlm.nih.gov/pubmed/28284827.
5. Lippi G. Biomarkers of myocardial ischemia in the emergency room: cardiospecific troponin and beyond. Eur J Intern Med 2013;24(2):97–9. Available at: https://www.ncbi.nlm.nih.gov/pubmed/23182628.
6. Froom P, Barak M. Auto-validation of complete blood counts in an outpatient's regional laboratory. Clin Chem Lab Med 2015;53(2):275–9. Available at: https://www.ncbi.nlm.nih.gov/pubmed/25153407.
7. McFarlane A, Aslan B, Raby A, et al. Critical values in hematology. Int J Lab Hematol 2015;37(1):36–43. Available at: https://www.ncbi.nlm.nih.gov/pubmed/24690478.
8. Genzen JR, Tormey CA, Education Committee of the Academy of Clinical Laboratory Physicians and Scientists. Pathology consultation on reporting of critical values. Am J Clin Pathol 2011;135(4):505–13. Available at: https://www.ncbi.nlm.nih.gov/pubmed/21411773.
9. Crawford JM, Shotorbani K, Sharma G, et al. Improving American healthcare through "clinical lab 2.0": a Project Santa Fe report. Acad Pathol 2017;4. 2374289517701067. Available at: https://www.ncbi.nlm.nih.gov/pubmed/28725789.
10. Nwaru BI, Friedman C, Halamka J, et al. Can learning health systems help organisations deliver personalised care? BMC Med 2017;15(1):177. Available at: https://www.ncbi.nlm.nih.gov/pubmed/28965492.

11. Cahan A, Cimino JJ. A learning health care system using computer-aided diagnosis. J Med Internet Res 2017;19(3):e54. Available at: https://www.ncbi.nlm.nih.gov/pubmed/28274905.
12. The Learning Healthcare System, Workshop Proceedings, National Academies of Science, Engineering, and Medicine, March 2007. Available at: http://www.nationalacademies.org/hmd/reports/2007/the-learning-healthcare-system-workshop-summary.aspx. Accessed March 17, 2019.

Decision Support in Transfusion Medicine and Blood Banking

Neil K. Shah, MD

KEYWORDS

- Decision support • Transfusion • Prediction • Modeling
- Patient blood management

KEY POINTS

- Clinical decision support (CDS) tools applied with good design can greatly enhance patient blood management through optimizing ordering and providing concurrent tailored patient information.
- Prediction and modeling will have increasingly important roles in managing blood inventory and coordination at donor centers and transfusion services to prevent wastage and supply shortfalls.
- Decision support and prediction have powerful potential applications for side-effect detection and management in both donors and recipients related to transfusion.
- With improved standards for health care data sharing, such as Fast Healthcare Interoperability Resources and increased adoption, there is a trend toward centralization of CDS content and tools.

INTRODUCTION

Clinical decision support (CDS) can positively impact many facets of patient transfusion therapy from demand-based collections at the donor center to detecting transfusion side effects in recipients. Classically, CDS in transfusion medicine has focused on blood utilization to help providers meet restrictive transfusion practices; less blood was shown to be equivalent or better for most clinical scenarios in large, randomized controlled trails.[1] This article aims to broadly cover the salient points in transfusion and blood CDS, including published work and novel use cases. It begins with some foundations important to achieving success.

The key to CDS is great design and applicability to the workflow. CDS needs to have a high positive predictive value, meaning that the recommendation being offered

Disclosure Statement: The author has nothing to disclose.
Department of Pathology, Stanford University, 300 Pasteur Drive, MC 5626, H1402-G, Stanford, CA 94035, USA
E-mail address: nshah3@stanford.edu

Clin Lab Med 39 (2019) 269–279
https://doi.org/10.1016/j.cll.2019.01.006
0272-2712/19/© 2019 Elsevier Inc. All rights reserved.

labmed.theclinics.com

should apply to most if not all of the cases. One should aim for specificity over sensitivity because false positive scenarios can quickly lead users to begin ignoring the CDS for all future entities and contribute to the commonly loathed concept of alert fatigue.[2] The concept of the "five rights" of CDS[3] was popularized and is vital to achieving a high impact-to-interrupt ratio (signal-to-noise ratio) (**Table 1**). The "five rights" also broaden the scope of CDS from just alerts to test menus changes and peer comparison as tools within a larger change model; they also broaden the playing space from just the electronic health record (EHR) to considering ancillary systems, such as donor center management software and patient/donor facing portals and apps. In fact, the best CDS is one that occurs automatically in the background without user notifications. Examples include adding patients with high hemoglobin A_{1C}s to a closely watched diabetes registry[4] to allow for downstream bulk actions, such as more regular laboratory test follow-up or closer contact with a case manager.

PATIENT BLOOD MANAGEMENT
Transfusion Indications

Several programs have increased appropriate transfusion rates by simply requiring ordering providers to select a specific indication[5–11] of why a product is required as part of the product order with or without provider follow-up. Some have gone further in reenforcing single unit[6] transfusion over multiple as part of the order. Most of these interventions have not verified the chosen indication versus the patient's laboratory or clinical data. Interestingly, one study triggered an alert based on laboratory data if it did not match the chosen indication and found almost 50% to 60% discordance between chosen indication and recent laboratory tests. Nonetheless, most studies describe modest reduction in product usage between 10% and 20% and concomitant cost savings. Requiring an indication likely works through multiple ways: by serving as real-time education at order entry, by forcing providers to reconsider the transfusion decision, and simply by introducing the notion that their practice decision is being monitored or tracked (Hawthorne effect).

Table 1
The "five rights" of clinical decision support

Modality	Explanation and Perspective
Right information	Only present evidence-based support in applicable scenarios High heterogeneity scenarios are not ideal for decision support
Right person	Only present to the individual(s) most directly tied to the action A nurse, respiratory technologist, pharmacist, or resident can be the sole receiver instead of all team members A patient or donor themselves can receive information through portals and apps pertaining to preventative care or recruitment
Right format	In addition to alerts, consider changes to order sets, preference lists, and test menus to optimize user action
Right channel	In addition to the EHR, consider the patient portal, clinical team messaging applications, automatic registry creation for chronic disease, and e-mail for peer review and comparison
Right time	Offer support closest to the time of action and within the user's existing workflow and space

Data from Sirajuddin AM, Osheroff JA, Sittig DF, et al. Implementation pearls from a new guidebook on improving medication use and outcomes with clinical decision support. Effective CDS is essential for addressing healthcare performance improvement imperatives. J Healthc Inf Manag 2009;23(4):38–45.

Best Practice Alerts

Alerts or pop-ups (**Fig. 1**) are generally used at the time of ordering if a provider's order for a product is occurring when patient recent laboratory test values are beyond guideline-supported thresholds; alerts often act in concert with the transfusion indication requirement described earlier.[9,10] Important exclusions have to be built-in to avoid triggering alerts in urgent situations, such as massive transfusion, or procedural settings, such as the operating room. Red blood cells (RBCs) have been the focus of most concurrent tool and alerts[7,12,13] and typically inform an ordering provider to discontinue order placement if the patient's recent hemoglobin is greater than 7 g/dL (8 g/dL in some studies or select populations). Although the measurement of RBC use varied in the studies mentioned as well as in a meta-analysis of CDS tools,[5] the studies showed improvements in RBC usage with demonstrated cost savings. There are fewer studies looking at the use of alerts for plasma[10,14] and platelet transfusions. These studies show a similar decline between 14% and 18% of product usage. Alerts targeting plasma transfusion are built to trigger on patients with a recent international normalized ratio (INR) $\leq$1.6 to 1.7. Platelet transfusions have several thresholds depending on bleeding and impending procedure. Targeting patients with recent platelet counts $\geq$50,000 per microliter is a reasonable threshold because that count is sufficient for most procedures/surgeries and considered sufficient even for patients with nonsevere bleeding. The author is using this approach in an upcoming planned platelet alert with important exclusions built for neurosurgery, bypass, extracorporeal membrane oxygenation, and for those on antiplatelet drugs.

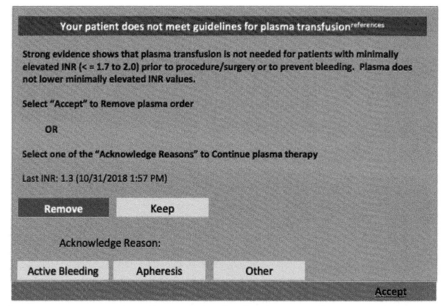

Fig. 1. Mock representation of best practice alert for plasma transfusion. This alert presents to providers in the author's EHR if plasma is ordered on a patient when a recent INR is less than 1.7. The provider can click "Accept" to remove the order or choose one of the acknowledge reasons as a clinical exception to continue the order. The alert is prebuilt with important exclusions to not trigger in apheresis, procedural settings, or as part of emergency and massive transfusion orders.

In place of alerts, some health systems have successfully used audits via transfusion technologists and residents[15,16] to discuss care with front-line providers to curb inappropriate transfusion. Although these systems can be effective, they require big investments of personnel time. The landscape of CDS is moving to more automated forms owing to the increasing sophistication of these tools and reduced resource requirements to build them.

Although interruptive alerts will continue to have some role in CDS, providers generally loathe them and consider any interruption of clinical care a nuisance. As such, alerts have to be a small part of an overall arsenal of CDS and must be well designed for specificity. In addition, small tweaks to their triggering mechanism can ensure that the provider is interrupted as soon as they select an inappropriate item rather than at the end at the time of signing after they have taken the time to fill out all order details.

Order Set Changes and Relevant Information Provision

Seasoned experts in CDS can attest that having fewer choices is better for standardized care. Removing inappropriate options or highlighting correct choices in order sets, formularies, procedure catalogs, and preference lists is very powerful. A second key observation is that users prefer helpful information alongside their work in the EHR rather than in interruptive forms that break their thought pattern. The following list (and in **Fig. 2**) shows several ways to modify ordering behavior to optimize appropriate transfusion based on order set revisions at the author's institutions and others.[2,17]

- Default single-unit orders for RBCs and platelets
- Limit the upper choice for RBCs and platelets in the quick pick list to 2 and require users some extra steps to order more (note: this does not affect massive transfusion orders)
- As part of product order placement:

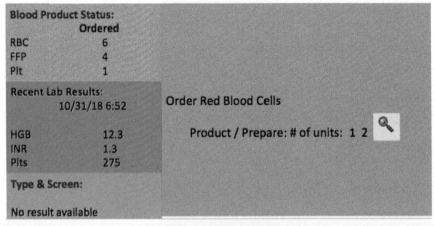

Fig. 2. Mock representation of blood product order screen. This is a sample of the blood-ordering screen in the author's EHR. Important changes have been made to promote restrictive transfusion practice. The single-unit order has been defaulted. A user has to go to the magnifying glass to search for units beyond 2. In addition, information on the left shows existing blood product orders to prevent duplicates along with recent laboratory tests to consider transfusion thresholds. Pretransfusion-required laboratory tests, such as type and screen results or lack thereof, are also displayed. FFP, fresh frozen plasma; HGB, hemoglobin; Plt(s), platelets.

- Provide tracking of how many units of different product types have already been ordered to prevent duplicate ordering by multiple care team providers
- Show recent laboratory test results, such as hemoglobin, INR, and platelet count
- Show relevant pretransfusion requirements, such as type and screen results
- Show anticipated blood loss and postoperative hemoglobin based on patient demographics, laboratory tests, and procedures

In addition to providing basic information that could be helpful on all patients, patient- and procedure-specific information to guide tailored therapy will be increasingly sought after as part of order placement CDS. Joint replacement procedures present one of the most common elective procedures, and models have begun to show increasing sophistication and accuracy to predict bleeding and postprocedure hemoglobin based on patient and surgical factors. Imagine being able to show an ordering provider this information and preventing transfusion or promoting single-unit transfusion to achieve the target postprocedure hemoglobin.[17,18] These models can be used in postoperative care[19] as well for more conservative blood use and/or quicker discharge of more stable patients.

Application of prediction models is not limited to RBCs. Achieving appropriate platelet count increment can be extremely challenging in hematology-oncology patients. Much of the underlying causes are patient related and nonimmune.[20–22] In addition, bleeding rates among this patient group are the same across a large baseline platelet count[23] (about 5K to 60–80K per microliter). Thus, it becomes far more important to transfuse those at highest risk of bleeding rather than simply increasing a platelet count to a certain threshold. Predictors of bleeding have been described, and there are novel descriptions of predicting a patient's response to platelet transfusion (platelet increment) based on patient and product factors.[24] The future of platelet transfusion should be guided by risk of bleeding and efficacy of transfusion rather than a count.

Peer Comparison

Comparing practice between different providers has been deemed to be a powerful way to curb outlier transfusion behavior.[5,25] In his experience, the author has found peer comparison to be extremely challenging and daunting from a lack of participation among different specialties. It will likely have a role as part of a broad change measure, and the following are provisions that are likely to add to success:

- Making utilization and regular review a departmental- or hospital-tracked initiative through leadership
- Automatic and regular dissemination of a dashboard or report to end users instead of requiring login or active action
- Greatly simplifying reports to a single summary page that can be digested in 10 to 20 seconds with detailed information available as needed
- Clustering providers with similar patient groups/operative procedures within a larger specialty
- Linking review and performance to financial incentives to align provider and system interests (within governmental and organizational bylaws)

Preoperative Anemia Management

A large focus of blood utilization has been to avoid or reduce use once the patient is in the hospital. Interventions aimed at optimizing patients hemodynamically before entry into the health system are woefully inadequate.[26] According to the World Health

Organization, about 10% of people over the age of 65 are anemic, and the number increases to 30% for those over the age of 85.[27] Patients who have elective procedures have higher rates of anemia[28] (20%–45%) due to underlying comorbidities. Preoperative anemia is an independent risk factor not only for increased likelihood of blood transfusion but also for increased perioperative morbidity and mortality. Duke University published an effective preoperative anemia management program[28] that coordinated care between surgical clinics, anesthesia clinics, and infusion centers. Although the numbers were small, the transfusion rate among referred patients was only 4% (1/25), and the clinic was able to demonstrate a large positive net present monetary value. A different publication tried a low resource-intensive measure in the form of alerts[29] targeted to participating surgeons for patients who could benefit from anemia treatment. Unfortunately, most alerts did not lead to therapy. Although facets of anemia management can likely be automated, a robust program would need coordination and widespread participation.

Future Trends in Blood Utilization

Two trends are noticeable in transfusion decision support. One is the use of several CDS tools simultaneously compared with stepwise approach. Most organizations have recognized that significant and sustained change requires a multifaceted approach that includes order set optimization, requirement of indications, concurrent patient-specific information, alerts, and peer comparison.

A more significant trend is toward centralization of CDS content and technology.

Key limiting reagents in uptake of CDS tools, especially for small health systems, are the lack of analyst build resources and the lack of knowledge of esoteric functionality within their EHR. These 2 factors were catalysts in vendors building out central repositories of CDS content. Vendors can extract relevant patient data from the EHR, process it through one or more algorithms on a central server, and return decision support back within the native system. A few other factors helping this centralization movement include the following:

- Better ability to update content knowledge and rule sets with change evidence
- Provision of comprehensive CDS that includes reports and peer comparison, alerts, and ordering usage statistics
- Greater expertise for validating advanced machine learning algorithms
- Increasing support for more facile health data transmission standards, such as Fast Healthcare Interoperability Resources
- CMS requirement for imaging decision support beginning in 2020

This centralization, however, is not a panacea. There are initial fixed costs, both monetary and time spent mapping and validating variables to existing data structure and ensuring that the knowledge presented is actionable. More importantly, gaining consensus and buy-in are the most challenging aspects of change, and this still is the primary responsibility of the parent organization.

DECISION SUPPORT IN INVENTORY MANAGEMENT

In addition to provider-side blood utilization, inventory management is important to prevent shortfalls/imports and more commonly to avoid wastage through expiration at the hospital or the donor center.

Inventory management is most challenging for products with a short life cycle. Thus, platelets naturally have been the target of frequent intervention. Some very simple strategies have been used to dramatically reduce outdates. A simple real-time dashboard at a multisite transfusion system[30] that showed inventory, patient product assignment, and current census of thrombocytopenic patients was able to reduce wastage by 40% relatively and 10% points absolutely. Another straightforward intervention that optimized operations and collaboration between the hospital transfusion service and the donor center[31] was able to reduce outdates from 19% to 9%. In this study, the findings from a consulting agency included logical and straightforward changes for both the donor center (collect more on Monday, less on Thursday, and rotate back platelets from smaller hospitals earlier) and the hospital transfusion (change weekday/weekend order-up levels and optimize platelet selection to prevent leapfrogging).

The field of more advanced decision support and prediction for blood product inventory modeling is nascent. Almost a decade ago, there was a stochastic dynamic programming model created that was combined with computer simulation[32] and showed that use of the system could potentially significantly reduce outdates and prevent shortfalls based on a small Dutch data set. Although this study model may suffer from general applicability, the examination of the blood product supply chain from a manufacturing inputs/outputs viewpoint is important.

A more novel approach to inventory management occurred recently by predicting near future platelet demand at a health system by training a machine-learning (ML) model with training data set comprising patient demographics.[33] It was found that certain characteristics were highly predictive of usage: weekday versus weekend, % of patients with abnormal complete blood cell counts, and the density of patient population in certain parts of the hospital. These predictors are intuitively logical (not always the case with ML models) because surgical loads are lighter on weekends, thrombocytopenic patients tend to use more platelets (likely more so if they are bleeding and anemic), and transplant/oncology patients are typically housed together. The model was shown to be able to reduce platelet wastage from 10.5% to 3.2% with high sufficiency built in to prevent shortfalls due to dynamic patient conditions. This novel approach would enable donor centers to collect based on a dynamic demand model from their supplied hospitals and could be trained and validated at different locations.

DECISION SUPPORT IN DONOR OUTCOMES AND HEMOVIGILANCE

Another growing area for application of technology and informatics is to actively monitor and predict donor side effects and transfusion reactions after infusion of blood products.

Managing Donor Side Effects

Vasovagal reactions are a common challenge at blood centers from both loss of donor goodwill and minor reactions to high risk and liability when a major injury occurs secondary to syncope.[34] Although early vasovagal reactions are commonly detected and treated at the donor center, late ones can be problematic. A center in Japan was able to identify features predictive of late vasovagal reactions by collecting demographics, collecting questionnaires, and exposing a small set of donors to a standing challenge for 3 minutes before and after blood collection.

Another common problem in donor management is the development of subclinical iron deficiency and reduced ferritin stores in recurrent donors. An institute in Germany attempted to find predictors[35] for developing subclinical iron deficiency by examining the ferritin level between first time and repeat donors, and second, by measuring several laboratory values prospectively on a small group of male donors at several time points after donation. They found that the hepcidin-to-ferritin ratio could predict what donors would regain iron stores by 8 weeks versus not.

Although these 2 studies are small, they illustrate the vast potential to use existing data, which is especially large now with donor center consolidation, to help drive decision support and prediction tools to optimize operations. Donors at highest risk for side effects can be preemptively identified and treated with tailored conditions, especially as more resources cannot be expended on all donors. They may even 1 day be used to determine which first-time donors are more likely to become recurrent ones or what day/time and mode of contact results in a successful donation.

Active Hemovigilance After Infusion

Several studies have shown that active surveillance for transfusion side effects and reactions results in a much higher detection rate[36–38] than passive mechanisms that rely on provider reporting. Examples of under recognized entities include transfusion-associated circulatory overload, or for reactions that can occur several hours after the transfusion, such as septic reactions from contaminated platelets. Effective and automated active surveillance systems are today rarely used because they require a great deal of design and validation to balance signal:noise. Nonetheless, with the aggregation of data in the EHR from multiple sources combined with increasingly discrete data storage, the future development of an automated and centralized hemovigilance system is possible.

SUMMARY

CDS has the potential to make EHR far more intelligent. CDS can empower coordinated, targeted, and efficient care by using underlying EHR data and freeing the clinician to pursue high order tasks independently and in concert with technology. This great potential will require prudence in applying CDS with thoughtful design such that it works nonintrusively with user workflows and provides specific and timely knowledge and action. It will also require a deep understanding of existing CDS tools and a mindset to absorb and pair novel ones on the horizon as summarized in the following:

- Patient blood management (PBM) and utilization remain important
- PMB works best through a multifaceted approach using ordering enhancements (transfusion indication requirement), best practice alerts, order set and preference modifications, provision of patient-specific concurrent information (existing blood orders and bleeding predictors), and peer comparison with ideally aligned incentives for provider and system
- Preoperative anemia management is an underappreciated treatment modality and can remove the need for transfusion and optimize patient outcomes
- Modeling and prediction have important roles in helping hospital transfusion services and donor center manage internal inventory, and importantly, coordinate supply to demand to limit wastage without supply shortfalls
- Decision support and prediction can be applied to manage transfusion side effects for both donors and recipients proactively while also 1 day optimizing donor recruitment and retention

REFERENCES

1. Carson JL, Stanworth SJ, Roubinian N, et al. Transfusion thresholds and other strategies for guiding allogeneic red blood cell transfusion. Cochrane Database Syst Rev 2016. https://doi.org/10.1002/14651858.CD002042.pub4.

2. Tim Goodnough L, Andrew Baker S, Shah N. How I use clinical decision support to improve red blood cell utilization. Transfusion 2016;56(10):2406–11.

3. Sirajuddin AM, Osheroff JA, Sittig DF, et al. Implementation pearls from a new guidebook on improving medication use and outcomes with clinical decision support. Effective CDS is essential for addressing healthcare performance improvement imperatives. J Healthc Inf Manag 2009;23(4):38–45.

4. Ali MK, Shah S, Tandon N. Review of electronic decision-support tools for diabetes care: a viable option for low- and middle-income countries? J Diabetes Sci Technol 2011;5(3):553–70.

5. Hibbs SP, Nielsen ND, Brunskill S, et al. The impact of electronic decision support on transfusion practice: a systematic review. Transfus Med Rev 2015;29(1): 14–23.

6. McKinney ZJ, Peters JM, Gorlin JB, et al. Improving red blood cell orders, utilization, and management with point-of-care clinical decision support. Transfusion 2015;55(9):2086–94.

7. Thakkar RN, Lee KHK, Ness PM, et al. Relative impact of a patient blood management program on utilization of all three major blood components. Transfusion 2016;56(9):2212–20.

8. Goodnough LT, Shah N. The next chapter in patient blood management: real-time clinical decision support. Am J Clin Pathol 2014;142(6):741–7.

9. Collins RA, Triulzi DJ, Waters JH, et al. Evaluation of real-time clinical decision support systems for platelet and cryoprecipitate orders. Am J Clin Pathol 2014; 141(1):78–84.

10. Yazer MH, Triulzi DJ, Reddy V, et al. Effectiveness of a real-time clinical decision support system for computerized physician order entry of plasma orders. Transfusion 2013;53(12):3120–7.

11. Saag HS, Lajam CM, Jones S, et al. Reducing liberal red blood cell transfusions at an academic medical center. Transfusion 2017;57(4):959–64.

12. Goodnough LT, Maggio P, Hadhazy E, et al. Restrictive blood transfusion practices are associated with improved patient outcomes. Transfusion 2014;54(10 Pt 2):2753–9.

13. McWilliams B, Triulzi DJ, Waters JH, et al. Trends in RBC ordering and use after implementing adaptive alerts in the electronic computerized physician order entry system. Am J Clin Pathol 2014;141(4):534–41.

14. Shah N, Baker SA, Spain D, et al. Real-time clinical decision support decreases inappropriate plasma transfusion. Am J Clin Pathol 2017;148(2):154–60.

15. Sarode R, Refaai MA, Matevosyan K, et al. Prospective monitoring of plasma and platelet transfusions in a large teaching hospital results in significant cost reduction. Transfusion 2010;50(2):487–92.

16. Marques MB, Polhill SR, Waldrum MR, et al. How we closed the gap between red blood cell utilization and whole blood collections in our institution. Transfusion 2012;52(9):1857–67.

17. Connor JP, Raife T, Medow JE, et al. The blood utilization calculator, a target-based electronic decision support algorithm, increases the use of single-unit transfusions in a large academic medical center. Transfusion 2018;58(7): 1689–96.

18. Huang ZY, Huang C, Xie JW, et al. Analysis of a large data set to identify predictors of blood transfusion in primary total hip and knee arthroplasty. Transfusion 2018;58(8):1855–62.

19. Trevisan C, Klumpp R, Auriemma L, et al. An algorithm for predicting blood loss and transfusion risk after total hip arthroplasty. Transfus Apher Sci 2018;57(2): 272–6.

20. Slichter SJ, Davis K, Enright H, et al. Factors affecting posttransfusion platelet increments, platelet refractoriness, and platelet transfusion intervals in thrombocytopenic patients. Blood 2005;105(10):4106–14.

21. Stanworth SJ, Navarrete C, Estcourt L, et al. Platelet refractoriness–practical approaches and ongoing dilemmas in patient management. Br J Haematol 2015; 171(3):297–305.

22. Uhl L, Assmann SF, Hamza TH, et al. Laboratory predictors of bleeding and the effect of platelet and RBC transfusions on bleeding outcomes in the PLADO trial. Blood 2017;130(10):1247–58.

23. Slichter SJ, Kaufman RM, Assmann SF, et al. Dose of prophylactic platelet transfusions and prevention of hemorrhage. N Engl J Med 2010;362(7):600–13.

24. Quaglietta A, Di Saverio M, Lucisano G, et al. Development of the Platelet Efficacy Score (PEscore) to predict the efficacy of platelet transfusion in oncohematologic patients. Transfusion 2017;57(4):905–12.

25. Zuckerberg GS, Scott AV, Wasey JO, et al. Efficacy of education followed by computerized provider order entry with clinician decision support to reduce red blood cell utilization. Transfusion 2015;55(7):1628–36.

26. Natera L, Roig XA, Rodriguez JCG, et al. Blood transfusion requirements in lower limb arthroplasties might be dramatically reduced if orthopaedic surgeons were concerned about preoperative anaemia. Eur Orthop Traumatol 2015;6(2):107–13.

27. Kansagra AJ, Stefan MS. Preoperative anemia. Anesthesiol Clin 2016;34(1): 127–41.

28. Guinn NR, Guercio JR, Hopkins TJ, et al. How do we develop and implement a preoperative anemia clinic designed to improve perioperative outcomes and reduce cost? Transfusion 2015. https://doi.org/10.1111/trf.13426.

29. Dilla a, Wisniewski M, Waters JH, et al. The effect of automated alerts on preoperative anemia management. Transfusion 2014;54(3):54A–5A.

30. Gomez AT, Quinn JG, Doiron DJ, et al. Implementation of a novel real-time platelet inventory management system at a multi-site transfusion service. Transfusion 2015;55(9):2070–5.

31. Fontaine MJ, Chung YT, Rogers WM, et al. Improving platelet supply chains through collaborations between blood centers and transfusion services. Transfusion 2009;49(10):2040–7.

32. Dillon M, Oliveira F, Abbasi B. A two-stage stochastic programming model for inventory management in the blood supply chain. Int J Prod Econ 2017;187:27–41.

33. Guan L, Tian X, Gombar S, et al. Big data modeling to predict platelet usage and minimize wastage in a tertiary care system. Proc Natl Acad Sci U S A 2017; 114(43):201714097.

34. Yoshida M, Ando SI, Eura E, et al. Hemodynamic response during standing test after blood donation can predict the late phase vasovagal reaction. Heart Vessels 2016;31(12):1997–2003.

35. Lotfi R, Kroll C, Plonné D, et al. Hepcidin/ferritin quotient helps to predict spontaneous recovery from iron loss following blood donation. Transfus Med Hemother 2015;42(6):390–5.

36. Hendrickson JE, Roubinian NH, Chowdhury D, et al. Incidence of transfusion reactions: a multicenter study utilizing systematic active surveillance and expert adjudication. Transfusion 2016;56(10):2587–96.

37. Hong H, Xiao W, Lazarus HM, et al. Detection of septic transfusion reactions to platelet transfusions by active and passive surveillance. Blood 2016;127(4): 496–502.

38. Agnihotri N, Agnihotri A. Active hemovigilance significantly improves reporting of acute non-infectious adverse reactions to blood transfusion. Indian J Hematol Blood Transfus 2016;32(3):335–42.

Technical, Biological, and Systems Barriers for Molecular Clinical Decision Support

Niklas Krumm, MD, PhD*, Brian H. Shirts, MD, PhD

KEYWORDS

- Clinical decision support • Genomics • Molecular pathology
- Electronic health record

KEY POINTS

- Clinical decision support (CDS) systems provide unique advantages for clinical use and interpretation of genomic data.
- Substantial technical progress in integrating sequencing data, interpretations, electronic health records, and CDS systems has been made in the past 10 years.
- Systemic and biological barriers remain comparatively unaddressed and are likely limiting the wide-scale and pervasive adoption of molecular CDS systems.
- A model for a hybrid consultative CDS system that integrates a genomics consultant with CDS systems may provide a path to overcome the remaining technical, biological, and systemic barriers.

INTRODUCTION

Over the past decade, high-throughput sequencing technologies have dramatically accelerated the capabilities and growth of molecular pathology. Concurrently with the rise of these sequencing technologies, the Health Information Technology for Economic and Clinical Health (HITECH) Act of 2009 created new mandates and incentives for implementation of electronic health records (EHRs).[1] These new incentives drove adoption of EHRs, with the goal of improving patient outcomes, decreasing costs, and increasing efficiency. Moreover, EHR implementation promised to centralize

Disclosure Statement: Dr N. Krumm and Dr B.H. Shirts are funded by the University of Washington, Department of Laboratory Medicine. Dr B.H. Shirts also receives funds from the Damon Runyon Cancer Research Foundation (DRR-33-15) and the Fred Hutch/University of Washington Cancer Consortium (NCI 5P30 CA015704-39).

Department of Laboratory Medicine, University of Washington, Box 357110, 1959 Northeast Pacific Street, NW120, Seattle, WA 98195-7110, USA
* Corresponding author.
E-mail address: nkrumm@uw.edu

and digitize vast amounts of patient data, enabling the creation of clinical decision support (CDS) systems.[2,3]

The advances in sequencing, her, and CDS capabilities promised to herald the age of precision medicine[4–7]—yet today, practical, wide-scale implementation of genome-enabled or molecular CDS remains seemingly distant.[8–10] In this opinionated review, how the field of pathology and informatics has approached, or failed to approach, the technical, biological, and systems barriers to adoption of molecular pathology CDS is explored.

CLINICAL DECISION SUPPORT FOR MOLECULAR PATHOLOGY

CDS encompasses a wide range of possible systems and contexts, many of which are not necessarily focused on molecular pathology or genomic medicine.[11] Within molecular pathology and genomic medicine, CDS typically has been implemented for medication selection and dose management[12,13] (ie, pharmacogenomics[14–16]), molecular oncology diagnostics and treatment,[17,18] laboratory order selection and support,[19] and/or prevention of duplicate or unnecessary germline testing.[20]

Motivation for CDS implementation within the broader medical context typically includes the standardization of care, encouraging evidence-based care[21] and ensuring that high-value clinical entities (eg, sepsis) are not missed. Reasons for implementing CDS for molecular pathology, however, are typically more specific and unique[22–24]:

- The scale of genomic information requires algorithmic interpretation and custom data presentation.
- Rapid advancement of knowledge and technological development within the field of molecular pathology creates opaque and rapidly changing test menus.
- Molecular pathology is not classically within scope of most physicians' training.
- The unique fact that genomic data is acquired once but has lifetime value (and can interpreted multiple times).
- Rapid technological development creating opaque and rapidly changing test menus

As within other clinical domains, the implementation of molecular CDS can be categorized into passive, semiactive, and active systems.[25] Passive CDS systems are simply knowledge bases, potentially tailored to a specific application and with an emphasis on clinical support. An example of a molecular passive CDS is a link to the PharmGKB pharmacogenomics database.[26,27] Clinicians and users of a passive CDS must be made aware of its existence but no specific workflows are required for their use.

As an extension of passive CDS, semiactive CDS systems provide links to knowledge bases and/or other decision support resources from within specific clinical workflows or triggers.[28] A molecular example is a drug-specific or variant-specific link to PharmGKB that appears when a provider orders drugs where pharmacogenetics are relevant. One common implementation of this type of system are info buttons displayed next to or nearby EHR result fields, order entry windows, or other components of a clinical workflow.[29] These buttons are configured to link to relevant and specific resources within passive CDS knowledge bases. The advantage of such a system is that detailed and relevant CDS is available to the provider on demand and does not interrupt clinical workflow; conversely, providers may not always recognize that information is available or that their specific clinical scenario may benefit from additional decision support.

In contrast to passive and semiactive systems, active CDS interrupts or otherwise manages the clinical workflow to ensure that relevant information is viewed or acted on. A molecular example is an alert that asks a provider to modify an order for drug when a patient has previously tested positive for a pharmacogenetic variant that is relevant to the ordered drug. Typical implementations of active CDS include pop-ups, which alert providers of particular patient characteristics, laboratory results, or order specifics. Other forms may include automatic order generation or modification, note template generation, messaging, or modification of result displays.

TECHNICAL DESIDERATA AND PROGRESS

Early CDS development in the late 1990s focused on the development of knowledge bases and databases to support passive molecular CDS (eg, OMIM[30] and PharmGKB[27]). By the late 2000s, however, it was recognized that passive CDS systems were not well suited for the growing size and complexity of genomic data and that operationalizing the delivery of CDS within clinical care would require additional integration.[31–33] In a seminal work,[34] Hoffman identified several challenges presented by the "genome-enabled electronic medical record" well before the introduction modern genomic sequencing technologies; remarkably, these challenges remain relevant today:

1. EHRs are optimized to access diagnostic results of transient value; genomic results, however, have lifelong value.
2. Data formats, vocabularies, and results need to be standardized to enable applications capable of enhancing clinical care.
3. Support must be enabled for periodic review and reinterpretation of previous genomic results as knowledge of underlying genomics and clinical significance evolves.

In 2012, Masys and colleagues[35] published 7 "technical desiderata" for the integration of genomic data into the EHR. These "desirable functional characteristics" defined how genomic data were to be generated, stored, transformed, viewed, and interpreted in the clinical realm. Noting that the initial 7 desiderata were likely insufficient for fully specifying the use of genomic data for CDS, Welch and colleagues[36] proposed an additional 7 desiderata for the integration of genomic data with CDS systems. These additional points primarily focused on the function and role of variant classification and CDS knowledge as well as the need to be able to scale the number of genes, variants, and connected CDS and EHR systems.

As an aid to the reader, the 14 technical desiderata proposed by Masys and colleagues[35] and extended by Welch and colleagues[36] are grouped into 4 major domains (**Table 1**; bracketed numbers refer to original numbering of desiderata):

- Systems should maintain a separation of concerns between data, interpretations, EHRs, and CDS systems [1, 5, 9].
- Systems should store data and associated metadata in a lossless format for the life of the data and/or patient but should transmit only the minimum amount required for function [2, 3, 4, 14].
- Systems should be capable of sharing data, interpretations, ontologies, and other layers using standardized and compatible formats [7, 10, 12, 13].
- Systems should be scalable and capable of many-to-many relationships between all levels; individual results, variants, patients, and interpretations should not be tied together in a fixed 1-to-1 relationship [6, 8, 11].

The authors emphasize that these desiderata may not be absolutely necessary for genomic CDS; rather, they represent a set of desired features. Many genomic CDS systems can be (and have been) implemented; however, reviewing the desiderata does provide a framework for assessing the advances and development since their proposal.

Table 1 Summary of proposed technical desiderata	
Systems should maintain a separation of concerns between data, interpretations, EHRs, and CDS systems.	• Maintain separation of primary molecular observations from the clinical interpretations of those data [1]. • Simultaneously support human-viewable formats and machine-readable formats to facilitate implementation of decision support rules [5]. • Keep CDS knowledge separate from variant classification [9].
Systems should store data and associated metadata in a lossless format for the life of the data and/or patient but should transmit only the minimum amount required for function.	• Support lossless data compression from primary molecular observations to clinically manageable subsets [2]. • Maintain linkage of molecular observations to the laboratory methods used to generate them [3]. • Support compact representation of clinically actionable subsets for optimal performance [4]. • Access and transmit only the genomic information necessary for CDS [14].
Systems should be capable of sharing data, interpretations, ontologies, and other layers using standardized and compatible formats.	• Support both individual clinical care and discovery science [7]. • CDS knowledge must have the capacity to support multiple EHR platforms with various data representations with minimal modification [10]. • Leverage current and developing CDS and genomics infrastructure and standards [12]. • Support a CDS knowledge base deployed at and developed by multiple independent organizations [13].
Systems should be scalable, and capable of many-to-many relationships between all levels; individual results, variants, patients, and interpretations should not be tied together in a fixed 1-to-1 relationship.	• Anticipate fundamental changes in the understanding of human molecular variation [6]. • CDS knowledge must have the potential to incorporate multiple genes and clinical information [8]. • Support a large number of gene variants while simplifying the CDS knowledge to the extent possible [11].

Bracketed numbers denote original numbering of desiderata by Masys and colleagues[35] and Welch and colleagues.[36]

Separation of Concerns

A core emphasis of the desiderata is to maintain separation between underlying sequencing data, associated variant interpretation, reporting EHRs, and interfaced CDS systems. Separation between these components is critical to allow for reinterpretation of primary sequencing data and sharing of data at either high or low levels (ie, interpreted variants vs raw sequencing data) as well as the ability to interface downstream systems (eg, EHRs).

Several different technical concepts can be used to support this separation, including service-based architectures,[36,37] a layered data approach, and/or the clinical standard reference genome.[35] Many of these approaches are concurrently aimed at mitigating the dramatically increased storage requirements of high-throughput genomics, because the current storage architectures of laboratory information systems (LISs) and EHRs cannot support storage of underlying sequencing data (discussed later).

In practice, complete separation between layers is difficult to achieve. In most clinical laboratories, raw sequencing data typically are kept on storage and compute infrastructure separate from the LIS and EHR. Most LISs/EHRs, however, are then sent static variant interpretations at a single point in time, usually in PDF format, which potentially combine multiple variants into 1 reportable result.[32,38] This arrangement reduces the technical storage burden on the LIS/EHR but violates several of the desiderata, including keeping underlying data and interpretations separate, as well as using only lossless data transformations. Furthermore, these reports are typically not in sharable or computable formats (discussed later).

A separate genomic data warehouse tightly interfaced with the LIS and EHR may represent another plausible solution.[31,38,39] This architecture keeps raw data, variants, and interpretations as separate but linked elements, which then can be independently referenced or transmitted to the LIS and EHR. This model may not be consistent, however, with the current Clinical Laboratory Improvement Amendments (CLIA) and Food and Drug Administration (FDA) reporting frameworks, where the clinical laboratory director takes responsibility for both the data and the interpretation. This framework may be one reason why the source of genetic data currently is the largest determinant of how genomic data flows into the EHR, rather than the content or use of the data.[40]

The genomic warehouse approach is not limited by the EHR's storage infrastructure but does impose new challenges in terms of workflow integration and results display. Laboratories supporting genomic assays and workflows may already have variant databases to support internal annotation and prioritization of variants. Typically, however, these databases may have unvalidated variant calls and do not meaningfully interface with EHRs, so they continue to rely on the production of static reports or single point-in-time interpretations. Tight integration of EHRs with genomic data warehouses remains a challenging barrier.

Data Storage Considerations

In parallel with the separation of concerns, the desiderata make specific recommendations that genomic data processing and storage solutions should support lossless compression, while also transmitting only the necessary information between systems and components. Advances in storage formats optimized for genomic data as well as the availability of scalable cloud storage solutions have provided plausible paths forward for lossless (or minimally lossy) data storage.[41–45]

Standards and protocols for transmitting the minimum set of data required are being actively developed.[46] The required amount and detail transmitted between external data warehouse(s) and the LIS, EHR, and CDS systems may vary dramatically. Currently, standards are being developed jointly by committees within the Health Level Seven International organization and the Global Alliance for Genomics and Health that specify how genomic information can be transmitted via the Fast Healthcare Interoperability Resources (FHIR) protocol. The Substitutable Medical Applications, Reusable Technologies (SMART) platform is being developed in parallel with FHIR protocols (SMART on FHIR) to facilitate apps using open standards for transmitting data for specific clinical use cases (discussed later).[47,48]

Use of Sharable Formats and Systems

Several of the desiderata from both Welch and colleagues[36] and Masys and colleagues[35] specify that genomic data and CDS knowledge should leverage open standards to support multiple EHR platforms, institutions, and contexts (eg, discovery science vs clinical care). Achieving these goals requires harmonization of ontologies and vocabularies, protocols, and developing standardized methods of extending EHR functionality.

Dozens of terminology systems and ontologies have been developed to describe clinicogenomic information, which has made integration of genomic data with EHRs and CDS systems challenging.[49] Nonetheless, several ontologies have now become de facto standards, including SNOMED, Logical Observation Identifiers Names and Codes (LOINC), and naming systems, such as International System for Human Cytogenetic Nomenclature (ISCN) and Human Genome Variation Society (HGVS).[50–52] More technically oriented formats, such as VCF, have standardized how sequencing data are processed and stored.[53] Encouragingly, these standards have had a synergistic effect on the development of additional standards, such as the FHIR standard, which are designed to specify and reference external ontologies. Furthermore, some systems have been developed that integrate representations of disease, gene, phenotype, and genetic test.[54]

EHR extensibility and integration has long been the Achilles heel of clinicogenomic systems, in part due to their custom and typically monolithic installation. Full-scale implementations of complete genomic CDS systems have been built, however, including their integration into the EHR. For example, 2 sites in the Clinical Sequencing Evidence-Generating Research (CSER) consortium developed genomic CDS approaches that could even potentially be implemented at other sites. In addition, several CSER sites built systems that delivered both structured and unstructured reports.[32]

Despite these successes, adoption of genomic CDS systems remains slow and challenging, because cross-site implementation is slowed down by hospital-specific or system-specific requirements and details. To address remaining challenges, there are now substantial efforts to develop app-like extensions to common EHR platforms via SMART on FHIR technology.[47,48] This platform will enable the integration genomic warehouse data into the EHR through a tailored data viewer. Sharing and dissemination of both warehouse data as well as the SMART on FHIR app will be enabled if both the EHR and the data warehouse use FHIR-compatible application product interfaces. This model can be further extended to include CDS systems, through the use of OpenCDS and CDS Hooks protocol.[55]

Scalability Issues

The last group of desiderata is focused on the scalability of genomic CDS systems. Welch and colleagues[36] suggest that CDS systems must be able to not only support the tremendous amount of existing genomic variation in the human population but also support multiple variants in unique combinations and haplotypes. The latter has become particularly important with recent advances in polygenic risk scores, where dozens or hundreds of variants are combined into a single interpretation.[56]

In addition to the scalability issues, there is particular emphasis in the desiderata on the ability to scale and adapt the relationships between sequencing data, variant classifications, and interpretations. Masys and colleagues[35] write that genomic EHRs must "anticipate fundamental changes in the understanding of human molecular variation," which they further specify as the ability to handle multiple genome-scale (eg, transcriptome and proteome) data sets over an individual lifetime. These data sets may be time specific, cell specific, tissue specific, organ specific, or disease specific; moreover, as single-cell technologies mature, these systems may be tasked with cell-specific or population-specific genomes. Although the authors believe meeting these requirements is feasible, to do so in a cost-effective way may require unprecedented collaboration between institutions on a national scale.[57] Significant additional work to define how these data are stored, accessed, and displayed remains.

BIOLOGICAL BARRIERS

Several biological realities make molecular CDS uniquely difficult to implement effectively. The most profound barrier is that there is still an enormous amount to learn. The current medical interpretation of any given molecular finding will have a relatively short half-life compared with the medical interpretation of many other diagnostics.[24] This would not be an issue if genetic tests were repeated as frequently as blood cell counts, but constitutional genetic findings are perceived to be relevant until death and maybe longer. Because of the paradox of long-lasting results with changing interpretations, optimal molecular CDS must be designed to access results stored indefinitely and pair these with current information (discussed previously).

The sheer complexity of human molecular genetics and the interpretation of genetic variation pose a second challenge. Gene-drug interactions, genes-environment interactions, and gene-gene interactions can be complex, and for almost every rule of molecular genetics there are exceptions. This complexity makes simple CDS rules difficult to implement correctly and difficult to operationalize at scale. Although larger data sets (eg, gnomAD[58]) have been instrumental in improving the ability to classify human variation, they have also put in perspective the magnitude of human variation. Every single nucleotide position that is compatible with life is almost certainly present in someone living on earth today. Thus, even at scale, a majority of discovered variants will be too rare for interpretations based on statistically sound, randomized trials, and instead their interpretations will need to rely on mechanistic or bayesian reasoning.[59,60]

Another limiting biological barrier is that evolutionary pressure has caused individual genetic variants with a large effect to be rare and allowed those with a minimal effect to become common.[61] This has a direct impact on the cost effectiveness and willingness to spend effort on genomic CDS efforts.[57] If there is a genetic cause for high morbidity or mortality, like malignant hyperthermia, it will be extremely rare. On the other hand, the genetic contribution of specific variants to common diseases, like heart disease and diabetes, is small. Interventions targeted at events that are both common and have a large health impact are obvious candidates for CDS, but evolution has ensured that any specific genomic CDS rule will never be in this category. Polygenic risk scores that combine the risk of many variants may be a counterexample to this principle, but the health care utility of these risk scores has yet to be demonstrated, and technical challenges for the implementation of polygenic CDS rules remain.

SYSTEMIC BARRIERS

Lastly, a set of systemic barriers to implementing molecular CDS systems is addressed. These challenges are potentially difficult to distinguish from technical barriers—because technical solutions are often seen to be the solution to systemic barriers. They are highlighted here separately, however, because their recognition is important to help guide the direction of technical development.

The Fragmented Nature of Medical Care

The current multiparty structure of the US health care system and systems in many other countries is a significant structural barrier to molecular CDS.[62,63] Sequencing data and variant interpretations for a particular patient will be spread across multiple institutions with different missions and business models. CDS rules may rely on the availability of variant data and/or underlying sequencing data (eg, through an external data warehouse) that has been appropriately formatted and validated. Patients may need to physically carry their sequencing data between systems then resolve issues of importing, formatting, and validating the quality of data to address issues of compatibility.

In addition to accessing the underlying data and interpretations, systems must be able to communicate when and why CDS rules were triggered and what clinical care actions were proposed and/or undertaken; for multistep CDS protocols, the state of the system also must be able to be transmitted when a patient transfers care. Currently, whereas some CDS-EHR integrations are able to automatically insert free text into clinical notes,[64] to the authors' knowledge, the ability to record and share the CDS system's state in a structured fashion has not been implemented.

Finally, issues surrounding identifying, accessing, and sharing familial genetic and health history information have not been fully addressed. As CDS rules become more nuanced and advanced, they may be able to act on data from related family members. These data, however, are typically entered as unstructured text and spread across multiple patient records.[65–67] Integration of data across related family members imposes additional challenges, including how family members will be uniquely identified and matched, if sharing of the data is desired and if approval to share data has been documented (even if the exact uses of the data may not be known at the time of sequencing).

Regulatory, Cost, and Reimbursement Issues

As CDS system implementations mature and become successful at their stated purpose (CDS), a new set of regulatory and oversight issues will arise.[68] These will be especially pronounced in light of the commonly touted advantage that CDS systems can overcome a relative lack of a provider's knowledge. The blurring of the lines between decision support and decision making will likely raise questions regarding which party (eg, the laboratory, informaticists, or end users) is responsible for medical errors that are traced back to the CDS system.[69–71]

The FDA role in regulating CDS systems has been evolving in recent years. In December 2017, the agency released draft guidance on its approach to regulating CDS systems and software[72]; in it, they called out several exempt applications of CDS but specifically identified software programs that "analyze and interpret genomic data" as remaining within the realm of FDA oversight. Although certain CDS systems may be exempted from FDA oversight, it seems likely that sufficiently complex CDS systems that draw on raw sequencing data, interpret multiple variants, and/or create polygenic risk scores will be considered as medical devices subjected to regulation.

Until recently, the cost of building molecular CDS systems has not been explored in depth. Using a local institution's experience in developing CDS rules for genomic results, Mathias and colleagues[57] analyzed the "cost per useful CDS alert" in a 1-way sensitivity analysis. Given the current state of sequencing costs, total patients sequenced, cost to build and maintain CDS rules in EHR system(s), and the probability that a rule will benefit a patient, the analysis finds that each triggered actionable alert costs approximately $4600. This analysis finds that with expanded scope and the economics of scale, the price per alert drops; however, only by having a large cohort of patients with sequence data at many institutions that share CDS knowledge does the per-alert cost drop below $100.

In addition to the high costs currently required to build genomic CDS systems, reimbursement for genomic testing is lagging.[73] In particular, reimbursement rules established by the Centers for Medicare and Medicaid Services specify that interpretation of results may submitted for billing only a single time and that providers or systems cannot be reimbursed for reinterpretation of variants.[74] This rule enhances CLIA and FDA testing validation and reporting frameworks by financially binding genomic data with 1-time laboratory interpretation. As a result, the financial justifications for CDS systems are almost always tied to finding or predicting cost savings from other aspects of a patient's care. Finding savings that offset the total cost of a genomic CDS can be challenging and ultimately may deter or prevent CDS applications even with proved medical benefit to the patient or health system as a whole. Finally, as molecular CDS matures and institutions and systems begin to share both CDS knowledge and underlying genomic patient data, cost-sharing and reimbursement between institutions or clinical encounters may become a central issue.

A MODEL FOR OVERCOMING BARRIERS

Some of the technical, biological, and systemic challenges to implementing a molecular CDS system are summarized (**Table 2**). From a technical perspective, significant progress has been made since the first desiderata were proposed, and the authors are optimistic that additional progress will be made. By their nature, the biological and systemic barriers are likely to prove more challenging—whereas some may be solved via technological innovation, others are unlikely to give way, and molecular CDS systems must be engineered around them. This last section proposes that CDS for molecular pathology take on a hybrid consultative model and discusses how such an approach can pave the way forward past these structural and biological barriers.

The idea of a hybrid consultative CDS system is that progress toward a complete active CDS system will develop only when genomic interpretation is first perceived to provide benefit and then when it saves time and effort to provide this benefit. A CDS system that provides limited initial active guidance and then recommends consultation with a genomics consultant (eg, a pharmacologist, medical geneticist, or molecular pathologist) for further guidance is an important first step. The consultant can then determine if the genomic data to answer the question exists and are valid and useable for the clinical question. If they are, the genomic interpretation or reinterpretation and clinical recommendation are provided. Alternatively, additional testing may be recommended if clinically indicated. Most importantly, the effort for this consultation would need to be a billable activity.

Table 2
Remaining technical, biological, and structural barriers

Technical	Biological	Structural
• Systems should support strict separation of raw data, variant calls, and interpretations, while tightly integrating result display into downstream EHRs. • There is only nascent consensus and adoption of standards and ontologies such as FHIR, SNOMED, and LOINC. • No robust support for multiple genomes per patient (eg, across time) and/or multiomic data sets.	• Accurate interpretation of genomic variants is inherently difficult. • Interpretations may change as knowledge base increases. • There are few well-defined rules for interpretation and many exceptions. • The inverse correlation between effect size and population prevalence limits high-value actionable variants and CDS rules.	• Transfer of genomic and CDS data between health care providers is challenging in a fragmented and multiparty health care system. • The regulatory landscape is evolving, including possible FDA oversight. • No reimbursement for reinterpretation of variants from existing sequencing data.

Although the hybrid consultative CDS system does not directly solve all the challenges of genomic CDS, it does ease the path to implementation in several important ways.

First, from a technical and regulatory standpoint, the CDS system can be greatly simplified, because it no longer needs to be capable of and responsible for making fully automated decisions. At the same time, the results delivered by the genomics consultant likely will be more nuanced and better tailored to a clinical situation. This is of particular interest when attempting to define CDS systems that capture rare variants or other genetically complex scenarios, where fully automated CDS systems would require intricate decision systems and/or machine-learning approaches that present a new set of validation and testing challenges. Moreover, the consultation can draw on other aspects of a patient's history (eg, family history), which are not typically available within structured fields amenable to machine-based interpretation.

Second, a hybrid CDS model also has substantial advantages from a systems perspective. The cost to build new CDS rules or features is substantially less, because the role of genomics consultants is flexible and they can quickly iterate on strategies to improve results. Furthermore, designing the model around a consultative system creates the potential for a billable activity, which captures the value of the genomic (re-) interpretation. Finally, reinterpretation of available genetic data from outside institutions would be within the scope of current medical care (this approach would be similar to how radiology tests and imaging data can be transferred and uploaded into institution-specific PACS systems before being re-read by radiologists).

The proposed approach does pose some new challenges as well. A hallmark promise of CDS systems has been that they provide immediate support and are minimally disruptive to clinician workflow. In a consultative CDS system, decision support could not be delivered in real-time; however, the authors believe that many scenarios where complex CDS is useful, a several-hour delay may be acceptable. In addition, the proposed model requires an available trained expert to handle CDS requests. This specialty does not currently exist. Molecular pathology may be most likely to fill this role initially, although medical genetics, genetic counseling, and molecular pharmacology might also be capable of providing genomic consultations. Depending on organization size and structure, additional consultations may increase costs—although such increases may be offset by improvements in test utilization as well as directly billing for consults/interpretations delivered.

Placing a component of human review into a CDS system may be seen as a step backward. It may be an ideal a stepping stone, however, toward better and more useful CDS systems. Once a complex task has been defined as clinically useful and billable, the rationale for reducing technical barriers and enabling faster iteration becomes obvious. Genomic CDS will become viable from a cost and reimbursement perspective rather than being funded by potential cost savings. All of the tools and technologies developed for molecular CDS systems can be utilized in a hybrid CDS model, including tooling to support rapid interpretation, reinterpretation, and CDS tools for the genomic consultant. Ultimately, the tools developed to support genomics expert under the hybrid consultative approach may become useful tools for fully automated active CDS applications.

SUMMARY

The implementation of a molecular CDS system is challenging. The authors find that although not all technical hurdles have been overcome, there exist full-scale implementations of molecular CDS systems, and remaining challenges are being addressed through the use of newer interoperability standards and protocols. Biological and systems-type hurdles remain and have received comparatively less attention. They now pose the most significant challenges to wide-scale implementation of molecular CDS. The authors emphasize that identifying a viable reimbursement model as well as addressing how to overcome the increasing complexity and the rare-variant interpretation questions are critical unaddressed questions. The proposal to create a hybrid consultative model addresses some of these concerns, although it also will introduce new concerns (such as workforce requirements and scalability). The biological realities of human genetics cannot be changed, but the authors look forward to how further technical innovation and systems-based innovations will enable widespread molecular CDS for the benefit of patient health.

REFERENCES

1. Marsolo K, Spooner SA. Clinical genomics in the world of the electronic health record. Genet Med 2013;15(10):786–91.
2. Kruse CS, Kothman K, Anerobi K, et al. Adoption factors of the electronic health record: a systematic review. JMIR Med Inform 2016;4(2):e19.
3. Rothman B, Leonard JC, Vigoda MM. Future of electronic health records: implications for decision support. Mt Sinai J Med 2012;79(6):757–68.
4. Tenenbaum JD. Translational bioinformatics: past, present, and future. Genomics Proteomics Bioinformatics 2016;14(1):31–41.
5. Ashley EA. Towards precision medicine. Nat Rev Genet 2016;17(9):507–22.
6. Collins FS, Varmus H. A new initiative on precision medicine. N Engl J Med 2015; 372(9):793–5.
7. Hood L, Friend SH. Predictive, personalized, preventive, participatory (P4) cancer medicine. Nat Rev Clin Oncol 2011;8(3):184–7.
8. Bouaud J, Lamy JB. A 2014 medical informatics perspective on clinical decision support systems: do we hit the ceiling of effectiveness? Yearb Med Inform 2014; 9(1):163–6.
9. Osheroff JA, Teich JM, Middleton B, et al. A roadmap for national action on clinical decision support. J Am Med Inform Assoc 2007;14(2):141–5.
10. Salari K, Watkins H, Ashley EA. Personalized medicine: hope or hype? Eur Heart J 2012;33(13):1564–70.
11. Garg AX, Adhikari NKJ, McDonald H, et al. Effects of computerized clinical decision support systems on practitioner performance and patient outcomes: a systematic review. JAMA 2005;293(10):1223–38.
12. Kuperman GJ, Bobb A, Payne TH, et al. Medication-related clinical decision support in computerized provider order entry systems: a review. J Am Med Inform Assoc 2007;14(1):29–40.
13. Samore MH, Bateman K, Alder SC, et al. Clinical decision support and appropriateness of antimicrobial prescribing: a randomized trial. JAMA 2005;294(18): 2305–14.
14. Relling MV, Klein TE. CPIC: clinical pharmacogenetics implementation consortium of the pharmacogenomics research network. Clin Pharmacol Ther 2011;89(3):464–7.
15. Bell GC, Crews KR, Wilkinson MR, et al. Development and use of active clinical decision support for preemptive pharmacogenomics. J Am Med Inform Assoc 2014;21(e1):e93–9.
16. Overby CL, Tarczy-Hornoch P, Hoath JI, et al. Feasibility of incorporating genomic knowledge into electronic medical records for pharmacogenomic clinical decision support. BMC Bioinformatics 2010;11(9):S10.

17. Yu P, Artz D, Warner J. Electronic health records (EHRs): supporting ASCO's vision of cancer care. Am Soc Clin Oncol Educ Book 2014;34:225–31.

18. Bucur A, van Leeuwen J, Christodoulou N, et al. Workflow-driven clinical decision support for personalized oncology. BMC Med Inform Decis Mak 2016;16(S2):147.

19. Roshanov PS, You JJ, Dhaliwal J, et al. Can computerized clinical decision support systems improve practitioners' diagnostic test ordering behavior? A decision-maker-researcher partnership systematic review. Implement Sci 2011; 6(1):88.

20. Dickerson JA, Cole B, Conta JH, et al. Improving the value of costly genetic reference laboratory testing with active utilization management. Arch Pathol Lab Med 2014;138(1):110–3.

21. Sim I, Gorman P, Greenes RA, et al. Clinical decision support systems for the practice of evidence-based medicine. J Am Med Inform Assoc 2001;8(6): 527–34.

22. Welch BM, Kawamoto K. Clinical decision support for genetically guided personalized medicine: a systematic review. J Am Med Inform Assoc 2013;20(2): 388–400.

23. Castaneda C, Nalley K, Mannion C, et al. Clinical decision support systems for improving diagnostic accuracy and achieving precision medicine. J Clin Bioinforma 2015;5(1):4.

24. Shirts BH, Parker LS. Changing interpretations, stable genes: responsibilities of patients, professionals, and policy makers in the clinical interpretation of complex genetic information. Genet Med 2008;10(11):778–83.

25. Berner ES. Clinical decision support systems. In: Berner ES, editor. New York: Springer; 2006. https://doi.org/10.1007/978-0-387-38319-4.

26. Khelifi M, Tarczy-Hornoch P, Devine EB, et al. Design recommendations for pharmacogenomics clinical decision support systems. AMIA Jt Summits Transl Sci Proc 2017;2017:237–46.

27. Hernandez-Boussard T, Whirl-Carrillo M, Hebert JM, et al. The pharmacogenetics and pharmacogenomics knowledge base: accentuating the knowledge. Nucleic Acids Res 2007;36(Database):D913–8.

28. Aronson SJ, Williams MS. Genetics aware clinical decision support. In: Genomic and precision medicine. Academic Press; 2016. p. 205–15.

29. Teixeira M, Cook DA, Heale BSE, et al. Optimization of infobutton design and Implementation: a systematic review. J Biomed Inform 2017;74:10–9.

30. McKusick-Nathans Institute of Genetic Medicine. Online Mendelian Inheritance in man, OMIM®. Available at: omim.org https://omim.org/. Accessed October 15, 2018.

31. Van Allen EM, Wagle N, Levy MA. Clinical analysis and interpretation of cancer genome data. J Clin Oncol 2013;31(15):1825–33.

32. Tarczy-Hornoch P, Amendola L, Aronson SJ, et al. A survey of informatics approaches to whole-exome and whole-genome clinical reporting in the electronic health record. Genet Med 2013;15(10):824–32.

33. Bates DW, Kuperman GJ, Wang S, et al. Ten commandments for effective clinical decision support: making the practice of evidence-based medicine a reality. J Am Med Inform Assoc 2003;10(6):523–30.

34. Hoffman MA. The genome-enabled electronic medical record. J Biomed Inform 2007;40(1):44–6.

35. Masys DR, Jarvik GP, Abernethy NF, et al. Technical desiderata for the integration of genomic data into electronic health records. J Biomed Inform 2012;45(3): 419–22.

36. Welch BM, Eilbeck K, Del Fiol G, et al. Technical desiderata for the integration of genomic data with clinical decision support. J Biomed Inform 2014;51:3–7.
37. Dournaee B, Natoli J, Juneja G, et al. Improving performance of healthcare systems with service oriented architecture. InfoQ; 2008. Available at: https://www.infoq.com/articles/soa-healthcare. Accessed October 15, 2018.
38. Kho AN, Rasmussen LV, Connolly JJ, et al. Practical challenges in integrating genomic data into the electronic health record. Genet Med 2013;15(10):772–8.
39. Horton I, Lin Y, Reed G, et al. Empowering Mayo Clinic individualized medicine with genomic data warehousing. J Pers Med 2017;7(3):7.
40. Shirts BH, Salama JS, Aronson SJ, et al. CSER and eMERGE: current and potential state of the display of genetic information in the electronic health record. J Am Med Inform Assoc 2015;22(6):1231–42.
41. Muir P, Li S, Lou S, et al. The real cost of sequencing: scaling computation to keep pace with data generation. Genome Biol 2016;17(1):4731.
42. Numanagić I, Bonfield JK, Hach F, et al. Comparison of high-throughput sequencing data compression tools. Nat Methods 2016;13(12):1005–8.
43. Shabani M, Vears D, Borry P. Raw genomic data: storage, access, and sharing. Trends Genet 2018;34(1):8–10.
44. Langmead B, Nellore A. Cloud computing for genomic data analysis and collaboration. Nat Rev Genet 2018;19(4):208–19.
45. Dove ES, Joly Y, Tassé A-M, et al. Genomic cloud computing: legal and ethical points to consider. Eur J Hum Genet 2015;23(10):1271–8.
46. Siu LL, Lawler M, Haussler D, et al. Facilitating a culture of responsible and effective sharing of cancer genome data. Nat Med 2016;22(5):464–71.
47. Alterovitz G, Warner J, Zhang P, et al. SMART on FHIR Genomics: facilitating standardized clinico-genomic apps. J Am Med Inform Assoc 2015;22(6):1173–8.
48. Mandel JC, Kreda DA, Mandl KD, et al. SMART on FHIR: a standards-based, interoperable apps platform for electronic health records. J Am Med Inform Assoc 2016;23(5):899–908.
49. Warner JL, Jain SK, Levy MA. Integrating cancer genomic data into electronic health records. Genome Med 2016;8(1):113.
50. McGowan-Jordan J, Schmid M, Simons A. Iscn 2016. 2016.
51. den Dunnen JT, Dalgleish R, Maglott DR, et al. HGVS recommendations for the description of sequence variants: 2016 update. Hum Mutat 2016;37(6):564–9.
52. Deckard J, McDonald CJ, Vreeman DJ. Supporting interoperability of genetic data with LOINC. J Am Med Inform Assoc 2015;22(3):621–7.
53. Danecek P, Auton A, Abecasis G, et al. The variant call format and VCFtools. Bioinformatics 2011;27(15):2156–8.
54. Paul Rupa A, Singh S, Zhu Q. GT2RDF: semantic representation of genetic testing data. AMIA Annu Symp Proc 2016;2016:1060–9.
55. Kawamoto K. CDS-Hooks. Available at: www.opencds.org.
56. Torkamani A, Wineinger NE, Topol EJ. The personal and clinical utility of polygenic risk scores. Nat Rev Genet 2018;19(9):581–90.
57. Mathias PC, Tarczy-Hornoch P, Shirts BH. Modeling the costs of clinical decision support for genomic precision medicine. AMIA Jt Summits Transl Sci Proc 2016;2016:60–4.
58. Lek M, Karczewski KJ, Minikel EV, et al. Analysis of protein-coding genetic variation in 60,706 humans. Nature 2016;536(7616):285–91.
59. Shirts BH, Pritchard CC, Walsh T. Family-specific variants and the limits of human genetics. Trends Mol Med 2016;22(11):925–34.

60. Tonelli MR, Shirts BH. Knowledge for precision medicine: mechanistic reasoning and methodological pluralism. JAMA 2017;318(17):1649.

61. Manolio TA, Collins FS, Cox NJ, et al. Finding the missing heritability of complex diseases. Nature 2009;461(7265):747–53.

62. Shankar P, Anderson N. Advances in sharing multi-sourced health data on decision support science 2016-2017. Yearb Med Inform 2018;27(01):16–24.

63. Sorani MD, Yue JK, Sharma S, et al. Genetic data sharing and privacy. Neuroinformatics 2015;13(1):1–6.

64. Wright A, Sittig DF, Ash JS, et al. Clinical decision support capabilities of commercially-available clinical information systems. J Am Med Inform Assoc 2009;16(5):637–44.

65. Doerr M, Edelman E, Gabitzsch E, et al. Formative evaluation of clinician experience with integrating family history-based clinical decision support into clinical practice. J Pers Med 2014;4(2):115–36.

66. Welch BM, Dere W, Schiffman JD. Family health history: the case for better tools. JAMA 2015;313(17):1711–2.

67. Polubriaginof F, Tatonetti NP, Vawdrey DK. An assessment of family history information captured in an electronic health record. AMIA Annu Symp Proc 2015; 2015:2035–42.

68. Coalition's reactions to public comments on the voluntary industry guidelines. cdscoalition.org. Available at: http://cdscoalition.org/wp-content/uploads/2017/08/CDS-3060-Guidelines-Final-2.pdf. Accessed October 15, 2018.

69. Greenberg M, Ridgely MS. Clinical decision support and malpractice risk. JAMA 2011;306(1):90–1.

70. Fox J, Thomson R. Clinical decision support systems: a discussion of quality, safety and legal liability issues. Proc AMIA Symp 2002;265–9.

71. Kawamoto K, Hongsermeier T, Wright A, et al. Key principles for a national clinical decision support knowledge sharing framework: synthesis of insights from leading subject matter experts. J Am Med Inform Assoc 2013;20(1):199–207.

72. Clinical and patient decision support software. fda.gov. Available at: https://www.fda.gov/downloads/medicaldevices/deviceregulationandguidance/guidance documents/ucm587819.pdf. Accessed October 15, 2018.

73. Deverka PA, Kaufman D, McGuire AL. Overcoming the Reimbursement barriers for clinical sequencing. JAMA 2014;312(18):1857–8.

74. Aronson SJ, Clark EH, Varugheese M, et al. Communicating new knowledge on previously reported genetic variants. Genet Med 2012;14(8):713–9.

Decision Support from a Reference Laboratory Perspective

Brian R. Jackson, MD, MS[a,b,*]

KEYWORDS

- Decision support • Esoteric testing • Reference laboratories • Information display

KEY POINTS

- Reference laboratories are rich sources of esoteric test expertise. Clinicians would benefit from this expertise at the point of care, but historically it has not always been readily accessible.
- Laboratory decision support is best viewed broadly in the context of the diagnostic testing workflow, from the selection of a test to the review of results. Each phase presents a different set of opportunities to share knowledge with the clinician.
- Most of the engagement of clinicians around laboratory tests occurs within electronic health record systems. To be effective at delivering decision support, reference laboratories must develop capabilities to integrate into these systems.

INTRODUCTION

Of all domains in health care, laboratory medicine could be the one with the largest need for knowledge support at the point of care. Certainly, medical knowledge is expanding and changing in all areas of health care. But when the sheer number of different laboratory tests that are commercially available is considered, and the rate at which these tests are updated and replaced with new tests, laboratory knowledge needs are likely greater than their counterparts in radiology, pharmacy, and surgical procedures.

Much of the innovation frontier in laboratory medicine exists in what is often referred to as esoteric testing. Although the term, *esoteric*, is not particularly well defined, it generally refers to testing that is not widely available at the local laboratory level and thus is sent out to reference laboratories. In some cases, an esoteric test may be new to the clinical environment and may require specialized instrumentation and

Disclosure Statement: Salary support provided by ARUP Laboratories, which is a not-for-profit entity of the University of Utah.
[a] University of Utah, Salt Lake City, UT, USA; [b] ARUP Laboratories, 500 Chipeta Way MC933, Salt Lake City, UT 84108, USA
* ARUP Laboratories, 500 Chipeta Way MC933, Salt Lake City, UT 84108.
E-mail address: brian.jackson@aruplab.com

Clin Lab Med 39 (2019) 295–302
https://doi.org/10.1016/j.cll.2019.01.008
0272-2712/19/© 2019 Elsevier Inc. All rights reserved.

reagents that are not available in the form of a commercial kit on a major platform. In other cases, the order volume for a particular test is simply too low for it to be cost effective for a local laboratory to perform, especially after considering overhead processes, such as quality control and proficiency testing. The volumes of tests on a hospital laboratory menu generally follow a power distribution, such that send-out esoteric testing represents approximately 90% of the variety of ordered tests in any given year, despite often being less than 10% of the total order volume.

Given esoteric testing's disproportionate share of the available variety of tests, plus the fact that esoteric tests are more likely to be new and more rapidly changing, esoteric tests represent a particularly large and important domain of opportunity for clinical decision support. In most cases (certainly ideally), the scientists developing esoteric tests and the laboratory directors who oversee reference laboratories are rich sources of expertise in both the analytical science and the clinical science underlying these tests. Reference laboratories have an ethical obligation to share this expertise with the clinical community and to share it in efficient, easy-to-access, and easy-to-apply formats.

INFORMATION FLOWS FOR ESOTERIC TESTING

Unfortunately, the traditional operational and information technology models through which local laboratories interact with reference laboratories have created barriers to access to this supply of expertise. In most cases, physicians do not place test orders directly with reference laboratories but rather through their local laboratory. When an esoteric test order is received, the local laboratory then forwards the order to a reference laboratory along with the specimen. After completion of testing, the test result and associated interpretive information flow back through the same pathway in reverse, from the reference laboratory to the local laboratory, at which point it is forwarded to the ordering physician. Results are often communicated at this point by means of entry into the electronic health record (EHR). In many cases, Health Level 7 (HL7) interfaces are used for transmission of orders and results, thus improving the speed and efficiency of the process. This requires that order and result information be reduced to the least common denominator of the capabilities of the HL7 interfaces, the laboratory information systems (LISs), and the EHR. Essentially, order and result information is typically restricted to what can fit into fairly short alphanumeric fields. This by itself is a significant barrier to embedding decision support information into order and result messages. In theory, if a reference laboratory were to interface directly with an EHR, this might open up some additional flexibility versus passing orders and results through an intermediary LIS. But currently this is not a common architecture.

The good news is that as EHRs mature, standards are emerging that promise to facilitate a much richer set of interactions between EHRs and third-party software applications and content libraries. Fast Healthcare Interoperability Resources (FHIR) and open clinical decision support (OpenCDS) are 2 HL7-endorsed standards that can allow software external to the EHR to access relevant patient data from the EHR and then present decision support back to the clinician within the clinician's standard workflow. At the time of this writing, commercial EHR support for these standards is still limited. But in the future, these standards should allow reference laboratories to interface directly with the EHRs used by ordering physicians to provide ordering and interpretive support at the point of care.

HOW DO PHYSICIANS CURRENTLY ACCESS LABORATORY MEDICINE KNOWLEDGE?

When considering how best to provide laboratory medicine decision support within clinical workflows, it is useful to start by considering the various ways in which clinicians access this type of information. A survey of more than 100 primary care physicians asked which resources they used to overcome uncertainty in ordering and interpreting diagnostic laboratory tests.[1] The most frequently accessed resources (beyond the patient himself or herself) were e-references; 57% reported accessing online reference sources at least once per week for help with ordering uncertainty and 46% reported accessing online references at least once per week for help with interpretive uncertainty. Other cited categories included talking with colleagues, referring the patient to a specialist, and simply following the patient clinically. Sadly, the least frequently accessed resource was laboratory professional, with only 6% reporting at least 1 such contact per week for both ordering and interpretive help.

There are multiple possible explanations for why clinicians do not take full advantage of the expertise of laboratory professionals. The most charitable explanation might be the evolution of electronic workflows in health care. In the distant past, consultation with hospital-based specialists, such as radiologists and pathologists, was mostly in the form of face-to-face and telephone interaction. Pathologists came to the operating suite to discuss frozen sections, infectious disease clinicians came to the laboratory to review culture plates, care teams stopped at the radiology reading room during morning rounds, and so forth. In today's health care environment, however, these workflows have mostly disappeared in favor of purely electronic communication.[2] The time demands are so great that if information is not available on a clinician's computer, then the clinician is unlikely to pick up a telephone, let alone walk over to another department to get questions answered.

So how can laboratories and laboratory professionals realistically share their expertise with frontline clinicians? The answer lies in finding ways to insert laboratory knowledge into existing electronic clinical workflows. Ideally, laboratories should embed comprehensive electronic decision support into each phase of the laboratory diagnostic workflow. On the surface this might sound like an overwhelming challenge. Just as clinicians are busier than ever, so are laboratory staff and their medical directors. This is exacerbated by financial pressures by hospitals and health systems to keep staffing levels low and testing volumes high. Pathologists and laboratory staff simply do not have much free time to build decision support software; author, edit, curate, and maintain decision support content; and lead clinical governance teams to review and approve all the content over time. Instead, they must prioritize their effort to do only those aspects that cannot be done well by someone else.

The good news is that in a world of electronic workflows, both software and content are theoretically highly scalable. Laboratories should not have to build everything themselves; they just need access to high-quality, trusted decision support content along with the means to integrate it into their clinicians' EHRs and computers. This is a natural role for reference laboratories. Partly because of organizational size, partly due to dedicated information technology staff, and partly because of their large customer networks (often hundreds to thousands of customer laboratories), reference laboratories are well positioned to develop and distribute laboratory decision support tools.

TECHNOLOGY CONSIDERATIONS

The best way to think about decision support from a technology perspective is to consider all of the various information platforms that support health care delivery. The most obvious and dominant (as of the time of this writing) are the EHR systems. EHRs have become the dominant electronic platforms for clinical data capture and display within both inpatient and outpatient settings.[3,4] Beyond those core functions, there are also myriad other functions supported by software applications in modern health care settings, ranging from scheduling to asset tracking to finance, which vary according to the specific needs of a particular department or unit. Some of these applications may be embedded into the local EHR; others may be best-of-breed systems or homegrown applications. Beyond these lie a wide range of non-EHR communication platforms, such as landline telephone, cell phone, secure text messaging, and health care–specific messaging apps. There are also communication platforms and applications used by entities outside of acute care settings, such as those used by home health agencies and retail pharmacies. And there are communication platforms and applications used by patients and their family members, which can range from Google and Wikipedia to more health care–specific resources. All of these are part of the information flow of health care, and thus all are potential candidates for laboratory medicine decision support.

In almost all cases, these systems are managed by entities external to, and thus not under the control of, reference laboratories. An additional complication is that privacy and security concerns make hospitals and health systems understandably cautious about allowing external entities to have access to their systems. The number and variety of such systems, given that reference laboratories may have hundreds to thousands of organizations they support, adds much more complexity. For reference laboratories to interface successfully into these various communication platforms, then, will require a high level of interoperability, such as that promised by standards, such as FHIR and CDS Hooks.

WORKFLOW CONSIDERATIONS

The laboratory testing life cycle begins when a clinician faces a situation for which a test is potentially useful and ends when the clinician reviews and acts on the test result. In the middle lie several processes, many of which involve some form of decision making on the part of the clinician. All such processes should be considered for clinical decision support (**Table 1**).

PREANALYTICAL PHASE

The first step in the laboratory diagnostic workflow is test selection. This involves much more than just a single decision about which test to select. It starts with the awareness that a diagnostic test might be applicable in a particular situation. It also includes knowing which of a family of related tests might be useful. It includes consideration of the patient's specific characteristics that might affect both the decision to test and the choice of tests. Finally, it includes decisions about the time course of testing, such as the appropriate time relationship to a therapeutic event or previous test.

The electronic workflow during the preanalytical phase occurs primarily within an EHR's order-entry function, including order sets, and it can also include reminders that may occur within other EHR functions.

Reminders

Some of the earliest successful trials of clinical decision support involved reminder systems.[5] Essentially, these were alerts pushed to physicians. In principle, reminders can take many different forms, including paper messages. Commonly they are implemented in the form of interruptive EHR. Interruptive alerts, although powerful, need to be carefully tuned based on clinical context if they are to do more good than harm.[6] For example, reminder systems within the Veterans Administration health care system

Table 1
Examples of reference laboratory–supplied decision support

Phase of Testing Process	Example of Actual or Potential Reference Laboratory–Supplied Decision Support	Supporting Technologies
Prepreanalytic	Online test menu with modern search features, embedded within CPOE application	FHIR, interfaces into EHR ordering applications
Prepreanalytic	Interruptive alerts, delivered as third-party content libraries with supporting evidence base	CDS Hooks, OpenCDS, EHR alerting software
Prepreanalytic	Order sets with links to online resources	EHR order set tools
Preanalytic	Secure messaging platform that supports communication among reference laboratory, local laboratory, and ordering clinicians	Secure messaging platforms
Postanalytic	Reports with fully customized graphical result presentation along with well-formatted explanatory material	PDF, interface engines, document repositories linked to EHRs

in the 1990s were likely responsible for widespread prostate-specific antigen testing on patients who were unlikely to benefit.[7] Customization of the reminders based on age and health status would have reduced the number of excessive tests and also would have reduced the degree of cognitive interruption to physicians. Reference laboratories that wish to produce decision support in the form of reminder systems must address both the software challenges of accessing clinical information within EHRs and the organizational challenges of fine-tuning the alerts for optimal effect (discussed later).

Order Placement

Steps involved in placing a laboratory order through an EHR computerized physician order entry (CPOE) system include identifying a test to order, selecting that test, and providing additional information as applicable to accompany the test order. A user can search for a test using an EHR search engine or can select a test from a previously created order set.

The accuracy of a search engine can be measured in terms of recall and precision, which are approximately analogous to the clinical assay concepts of sensitivity and specificity. Mainstream Internet search engines, such as Google and Bing, are so reliable and so familiar that search reliability is often taken for granted by end users. But unlike the highly sophisticated algorithms behind major Internet search engines, EHR menu search engines often use simple string-matching algorithms that can easily miss tests and mislead users. For example, a search for "CSF cell count" could fail to return a test named "cytometry, cerebrospinous fluid" or vice versa. Similarly, in situations involving multiple related tests, the order in which those tests are presented to the user can have a large impact on which test is ultimately selected. For example, some systems present results alphabetically. In such a system, "vitamin D 1,25-OH" would display above "vitamin D 25-OH", creating a risk of erroneous ordering in the vast majority of cases where the 25-OH test was the appropriate choice.

Laboratory test menu search engines thus represent a powerful potential opportunity for influencing testing decisions. Most laboratories have online test menus, which are often provided and hosted by reference laboratories. In many cases these menus include modern search engine functionality and rich metadata, such as analytical methods, ordering recommendations, and other information that clinicians can use to clarify which test to order and when. From a user perspective, these are all familiar features similar to what is found on shopping Web sites. The key is to integrate these highly functional laboratory Web sites with EHR ordering tools. Although such integration is not currently supported by mainstream commercial EHRs, there is hope that this will be available in the future (discussed later).

In cases of more repetitive, routine testing, search engines are too time consuming for regular use. Clinicians, therefore, rely extensively on order sets, which typically combine commonly used laboratory tests together with common drugs and other interventions, in a format where the selection and ordering can be done much more quickly. Order sets present an additional opportunity for reference laboratory–based decision support in the form of order set content libraries. Most reference laboratories are unlikely to engage in the full spectrum of order set–based decision support, given the broad range of nonlaboratory orders typically present (medications, nursing, dietary, and so forth). But there can be opportunities for laboratories to partner with decision support content vendors to extend the range of laboratory testing knowledge available in their products.

PREANALYTICAL PHASE

The next phase of the laboratory testing process occurs when an order is received by the laboratory and reconciled with the physical specimen. This phase includes a critical quality-control function in ensuring that the order and specimen were obtained and sent properly. Not infrequently, ambiguities and errors are discovered at this stage. Most of these problems involve either the physical specimen or the information contained in the order. Specimen issues include identification of the wrong specimen type, wrong submission temperature, broken or leaking tube, insufficient sample for testing, and so forth. Information issues include discrepancies involving patient identifiers, missing clinical information, underspecified orders, and so forth.

Although many of these issues traditionally would not be classified as decision support opportunities, many of them require communication with the ordering physician. For example, in 1 reference laboratory–based study, approximately one-third of all genetic tests were found misordered.[8] These orders were corrected (usually by replacing a test with a more appropriate one) after communication with the ordering physicians. This type of ordering clarification thus lies on the continuum of clinical decision support. Today, much of this communication occurs by telephone, but secure text messaging platforms are emerging that promise to improve the speed and efficiency of laboratory-clinician communication. In cases of esoteric testing, where there can be several degrees of separation between the ordering clinician and the performing laboratory, the ability to communicate via secure messaging would be particularly valuable. Such platforms initially will be a means for human-to-human communication but will be a natural opportunity for embedding automated decision support in the future.

POSTANALYTICAL PHASE

Once a test result is verified, the postanalytical phase consists of delivery of the result to the provider and the medical record. The key decisional task, and thus the decision support opportunity, is in proper interpretation of the test result in the context of the particular patient scenario. This includes decisions about any diagnostic and/or therapeutic actions to be taken based on the test result.

The natural location for interpretive decision support is directly adjacent to the test result, that is, embedded in the result display. This may sound simple but in practice presents several significant challenges. Classically, test results were delivered in the form of paper reports, and this format is still widely used in the laboratory industry. In cases of a reference laboratory sensing a report document directly to an ordering clinician, the laboratory can in principle use a combination of explanatory text, tables, and/or figures to communicate the nuances of the test and result. In many cases, however, reference laboratory reports only make it as far as the local laboratory, where the results are transcribed into an LIS. Paper report formats are thus limited as a reference laboratory communication tool. One way to extend the utility of document-based reports is to deliver them electronically, for example, as portable document format (PDF) files, which can be downloaded by clinicians and also be transmitted via established interfaces into document management systems and EHRs.[9]

On the other hand, most laboratory results are currently viewed not in the form of documents but rather in the form of spreadsheets and lists within EHR applications. The ability of humans to quickly and intuitively interpret data is highly dependent on the visual presentation of that data.[10] Display formats that are reasonable and appropriate for some tests, for example, routine chemistry panels, may be highly inadequate for more complex esoteric tests. Unfortunately, the visual presentation is under the control of the EHR software and not the performing laboratory. Emerging standards, such as FHIR, might in the future open up opportunities for reference laboratories to customize result display within EHRs.

GOVERNANCE

An often underappreciated component of clinical decision support is governance. Modern medicine involves an incredibly complex set of activities. Although clinical decision support might seem on the surface to be a straightforward process of providing evidence-based guidance to clinicians, in practice there are several subtleties that can determine its level of success.

Consider that decision support is fundamentally a means of managing clinicians. As with most management activities, the best managers are those who are close to the people being managed and understand the nuances and complexities of the local environment. In cases of the practice of medicine, the ideal managers of clinicians are those who work in the same institution, have clinical backgrounds, and can collaborate with their frontline clinician peers to fine-tuning processes in pursuit of the better outcomes. Unfortunately, many decision support efforts have been driven at the level of large insurance companies, accreditation bodies, and regulatory agencies. Although such organizations can certainly play a supporting role in encouraging decision support and removing barriers to its implementation, there are serious risks to implementing specific rules at such a high level. Regulatory agencies, accreditation bodies, and payers are removed from the details of frontline care, which can lead to unintended consequences when they attempt to enforce particular aspects of decision support.

Reference laboratories are likewise organizationally separate from the point of care and are thus subject to some of the same risks as regulatory bodies and payers. A key to success is in ensuring an appropriate division of labor: reference laboratories are well positioned to perform knowledge curation and software development, but the fine-tuning, monitoring, and ultimate control belong in the hands of the local clinical organization.

SUMMARY

Esoteric testing presents a broad range of opportunities to improve clinical decision making. To be effective, the knowledge support needs to be seamlessly embedded into clinical workflows. Reference laboratories are uniquely positioned to play an outsized role in laboratory decision support, in part because they are large repositories of esoteric testing knowledge and in part because of their resources and client relationships. To accomplish this, however, reference laboratories must develop strong capabilities to integrate content and logic into clinical software platforms, including but not limited to EHRs.

REFERENCES

1. Hickner J, Thompson PJ, Wilkinson T, et al. Primary care physicians' challenges in ordering clinical laboratory tests and interpreting results. J Am Board Fam Med 2014;27(2):268–74.
2. Wachter R. The digital doctor: hope, hype, and harm at the dawn of medicine's computer age. New York: McGraw Hill; 2015.
3. Arndt BG, Beasley JW, Watkinson MD, et al. Tethered to the EHR: primary care physician workload assessment using EHR event log data and time-motion observations. Ann Fam Med 2017;15(5):419–26.
4. Sinsky C, Colligan L, Li L, et al. Allocation of physician time in ambulatory practice: a time and motion study in 4 specialties. Ann Int Med 2016;165:753–60.
5. McDonald CJ, Overhage JM, Tierney WM, et al. The regenstrief medical record system: a quarter century experience. Int J Med Inform 1999;54(3):225–53.
6. Powers EM, Shiffman RN, Melnick ER, et al. Efficacy and unintended consequences of hard-stop alerts in electronic health record systems: a systematic review. J Am Med Inform Assoc 2018;25(11):1556–66.
7. Walter LC, Bertenthal D, Lindquist K, et al. PSA screening among elderly men with limited life expectancies. JAMA 2006;296(19):2336–42.
8. Miller CE, Krautscheid P, Baldwin EE, et al. Genetic counselor review of genetic test orders in a reference laboratory reduces unnecessary testing. Am J Med Genet A 2014;164A(5):1094–101.
9. Shirts BH, Gundlapalli AV, Jackson B. Pilot study of linking web-based supplemental interpretive information to laboratory test reports. Am J Clin Pathol 2009;132(6):818–23.
10. Tufte ER. The visual display of quantitative information. 2nd edition. Cheshire (CT): Graphics Press; 2001.

Training Aspects of Laboratory-Based Decision Support

Bruce P. Levy, MD[a,b,*]

KEYWORDS

- Decision support • Clinical pathology informatics
- Undergraduate medical education • Pathology residency • Pathology fellowships
- Continuing medical education • Educational electronic health record

KEY POINTS

- Informatics and clinical decision support (CDS) is an important part of the daily practice of pathology and medicine.
- Education in CDS must be part of a broader educational program in clinical and pathology informatics.
- CDS and informatics should be an educational thread from the first day of medical school through continuing medical education.
- The education should be practical and outcomes based, and use educational versions of electronic clinical systems to support exercises and simulations.

INTRODUCTION

Clinical decision support (CDS) tools are designed to assist physicians and other health professionals in making appropriate clinical decisions in a variety of situations. Properly designed and implemented, CDS should effectively and efficiently provide clinicians with needed medical intelligence at the appropriate time and with minimal disruption to their workflow. CDS has been extensively used for several years in assisting physicians in the ordering of appropriate laboratory tests.[1–3] CDS is being increasingly used in assisting physicians in the interpretation of laboratory results and recommendations regarding additional testing and/or treatment options,[4,5] and there are additional opportunities in patient-facing CDS for interpretation of laboratory tests.[6]

CDS tools are not without controversy and issues that can make these tools more of a nuisance for providers. A significant percentage of CDS alerts are overridden by

Disclosure Statement: The author has nothing to disclose.
[a] Education and Research, Geisinger Health, 100 North Academy Avenue, MC 30-39, Danville, PA 17822, USA; [b] Geisinger Commonwealth School of Medicine, 525 Pine Street, Scranton, PA 18509, USA
* 100 North Academy Avenue, MC 30-39, Danville, PA 17822.
E-mail address: blevy2@geisinger.edu

providers for a variety of reasons that include alert fatigue, usability issues, workflow disruptions, and differing professional opinions regarding existing guidelines.[7,8] For laboratory test ordering, CDS has been shown to have minimal effect on compliance, but no significant impact on clinical outcomes that would recommend their increased use,[9,10] despite long-standing recommendations for effective CDS such as the "Ten Commandments" of CDS.[11]

Pathologists and the laboratory's technical leadership have historically had minimal input in the development of CDS tools that affect test ordering, which has been designed and implemented by the health system's information technology teams, with or without the support of physician informaticians. As a result, many of these CDS tools may not meet the needs of our clinicians and pathologists, and therefore inadequately serve our patients. Examples of where pathology departments have had either input in or control over laboratory-directed CDS tool creation do exist, and demonstrate the value that pathology can provide in the design, development, implementation, and analysis of CDS related to laboratory test ordering and result interpretation.[12-14]

As CDS involving laboratory testing becomes pervasive and expands into the area of laboratory result analysis and interpretation, the need for the expertise of pathologists and technical leadership in the design and development of laboratory-related CDS tools gains increasing importance. Pathologists have not only unique clinical and diagnostic expertise but also years of experience in working with their laboratory information systems to generate and analyze data to drive increased laboratory quality and efficiency.[15] Although most pathologists, whether recognized or not, have some knowledge of pathology informatics, there is a significant gap in their knowledge of CDS tools and other aspects of clinical informatics. This is not solely the responsibility of pathology and its training programs, but is just one part of the greater deficiency in informatics education and training for physicians and other health professionals.

The challenge facing pathology is to provide sufficient education and training for our pathologists and laboratory management in the design, development, implementation, and analysis of laboratory-related CDS tools. This must be incorporated into a broader curriculum for training in clinical and pathology informatics. Although pathology has taken some leadership in this area through the incorporation of informatics into the program requirements for Accreditation Council for Graduate Medical Education (ACGME)-accredited residency programs in pathology, board examinations in pathology, and the development of Pathology Informatics Essential for Residents (PIER), there remains much work ahead.[16-18] At the same time, a more concerted effort toward providing an educational foundation in informatics for all physicians and health professionals needs to be advanced.

This article is divided into sections by educational level, exploring specifically the current state and aspirations for education and training in the subspecialty of informatics and CDS. It is important that a strong background in the general principles of clinical and pathology informatics is a required prerequisite for adequate training in the creation and support of CDS tools. Also, it would be most advantageous to have informatics education run as a thread throughout medical education, from the first day of medical school through graduate and continuing medical education. Otherwise, the burden on individual training programs in pathology to provide all the necessary training in informatics and CDS will be considerable.

UNDERGRADUATE MEDICAL EDUCATION

For more than a century, most undergraduate medical education has been taught based on the educational system established after the 1910 publication of the Flexner

Report critiquing the then state of medical education in the United States and Canada.[19] As a relatively new subspecialty within medicine, informatics was unknown at the time of the Flexner report and had not been included in this traditional medical school curriculum. With an already overloaded curriculum locked into courses based on scientific topics of focus, it has been extremely difficult to incorporate any meaningful informatics education. There have been recent efforts to evolve the medical school curriculum to better reflect the needs of American health care and to prepare it for the future.[20] This restructuring of undergraduate medical education includes longitudinal experiences and disease- or organ-based education, and offers an opportunity to incorporate informatics education into medical school.

There is interest in clinical informatics education among medical students. A survey among University of Utah medical students suggested that informatics content in medical school is desired.[21] A survey of 4 United States allopathic medical schools that received responses from 557 medical students revealed that nearly 60% of medical students desired some informatics training opportunities in either medical school or residency.[22] These results are not surprising for a generation that does not remember a time without computers, smart devices, the Internet, or social media.

In the late 1990s, the Association of American Medical Colleges created the Medical School Objectives Project (MSOP) to better define learning objectives that medical schools could use as part of the evolution of medical education. One of the foci of the second report of the MSOP focused on medical informatics education, which was closely linked to 5 major roles played by physicians: lifelong learner, clinician, educator-communicator, researcher, and manager. The report went on to define specific informatics objectives that students should be able to accomplish in each of these roles and the knowledge that is required to achieve these objectives.[23] The American Medical Association, as part of Accelerating Change in Medical Education, awarded 11 grants to United States medical schools for the development of a new comprehensive health science curriculum for undergraduate medical education. A study reviewing all 30 of the grant submissions and the curricula developed by the 11 grant recipients identified clinical informatics as 1 of 6 core domains within the undergraduate medical education curricular framework, which was defined as "All issues related to the application of informatics and information technology to deliver health care services, including CDS, documentation, electronic medical records, and the utilization of data to improve health."[24]

In a 2007 to 2008 survey, 86% of United States medical schools reported that informatics was included as a required course.[25] It seems that many of these institutions have used a relatively broad definition of informatics with a narrow focus on the education, whereby education in library science and literature searching is the extent of the "informatics" education.[26,27] Although all physicians must have skills in identifying and critically evaluating the medical literature and applying the principles of evidence-based medicine, it should be obvious that this alone does not represent clinical informatics education.

The American Medical Informatics Association (AMIA) published a white paper defining the core content for the subspecialty of clinical informatics, in which they place clinical informatics at the intersection of clinical care, the health system, and information and communications technology. The core content is divided among the 4 major categories of Fundamentals, The Health System, Clinical Decision Making and Care Process Improvement, and Leading and Managing Change, and is further divided into individual topics and subtopics.[28] A similar effort within the pathology informatics community identified the 4 primary divisions of pathology informatics to include Information Fundamentals, Information Systems, Workflow and Processes, and Governance and Management. These were broken down into 96 individual topic areas that were to serve as the curriculum for fellowship training in pathology informatics.[29]

Whereas AMIA and the aforementioned pathology community work focused more on the entire breadth of clinical and pathology informatics, there has been some work on identifying the aspects of clinical informatics that every physician needs to know, including some suggestions for incorporating informatics into undergraduate medical education. The International Medical Informatics Association (IMIA) first published recommendations for informatics education in 2000, which were revised in 2010. Part of IMIA's efforts identified which aspects of informatics are applicable to undergraduate medical education.[30,31] This approach was applied in Germany, where there has been more than 4 decades of informatics education for German medical students.[32]

In the United States, there has been interest in incorporating informatics education into medical school. As part of Curriculum 2000, the University of Alabama proposed an approach to informatics education for medical students that focused on physicians functioning as information managers. Among other competencies, they specifically identified decision analysis and decision support tools as required knowledge.[33] The University of Vermont College of Medicine described a 4-year integrated curriculum in information literacy and applied medical informatics that suggested integrating informatics throughout the medical school curriculum and including "information faculty" into the teaching team.[34]

The University of Arizona College of Medicine established a Biomedical Informatics (BMI) curriculum as part of its new medical school campus in Phoenix in 2007. BMI was identified as a longitudinal theme across the integrated system blocks in the first 2 years of medical school, whereby appropriate informatics skills were integrated into the blocks as appropriate. A BMI block was created to provide specific informatics knowledge such as data privacy/security and CDS tools. The content and delivery evolved over time with feedback from students, experience in teaching, and in response to budgetary pressures. They were able to compare the Phoenix students with Tucson medical students who did not receive the informatics curriculum, and noted significant differences in self-assessment scores between the 2 groups of students in some but not all informatics competencies.[35]

Oregon Health and Sciences University (OHSU) formed a group that identified key informatics competencies for physicians, which were mapped to the 6 ACGME core competency domains, as well as defining specific learning objectives and milestones for each competency. The competencies spanned informatics from basic information searching skills through knowledge of bioinformatics, population health, telehealth, and CDS. OHSU then identified at which time during medical education these competencies should be taught and discussed different methods for incorporating informatics into the medical school curriculum.[36] Some of the OHSU recommendations were incorporated into the Accelerating Change in Medical Education project.[24]

The Medical University of South Carolina (MUSC) described a project in which they educated and enrolled medical students in the creation of CDS tools. A second-year medical school course in evidence-based practice (EBP) was repurposed and focused on clinically relevant, process-driven projects in which medical students were partnered with clinical teams to create decision support tools. This education is reinforced during the clinical years with EBP projects in the internal medicine and pediatric clerkships. Feedback from students and faculty were positive, and adjustments to the program have been made on the basis of this feedback.[37]

The available medical literature clearly demonstrates that there is significant interest in and support for informatics education in undergraduate medical education among medical students and some medical school faculties. CDS is a commonly recognized aspect of this training. It has also been demonstrated that there are several obstacles to the implementation of informatics education in medical school, including lack of time to engage with students within the existing medical curriculum, uncertainty among faculty as to their ability and bandwidth to teach informatics, and a lack of consistent support among senior leadership at medical schools.

The key features of a successful educational program for informatics and decision support in undergraduate medical education include the following.

1. *Informatics as an educational thread.* Informatics, as a part of the daily practice of medicine, cannot be adequately taught in a single course or series of lectures. It must be incorporated throughout the medical school curriculum as a part of every applicable medical school course and rotation. It also needs to be integrated with informatics education at the postgraduate and continuing education levels.
2. *Informatics needs clearly defined objectives and outcomes.* The curriculum cannot be limited to a list of topics students need to know. Specific objectives with measurable outcomes at different educational levels must be developed and tracked.
3. *Use multiple educational techniques.* Informatics content should be delivered through a variety of methods and mechanisms. These include not only some traditional lectures, but also online learning, small groups, flipped classrooms, and practical exercises.
4. *Informatics is about doing, not just knowing.* Informatics education needs to be supported through exercise-based activities, such as the CDS tool-building exercise described at MUSC. These exercises should be incorporated appropriately throughout the curriculum, based on real-world scenarios, and should provide increasing sophistication as the student progresses.
5. *Informatics is a team sport.* Education and training in clinical informatics should not be restricted to doctoral-level individuals for either the students or faculty. Students should have the opportunity to work on their informatics projects in multidisciplinary teams and be taught by experts from clinical, scientific, and technical backgrounds as appropriate.
6. *Use of educational versions of clinical systems as an educational tool.* It is critical that medical students have the opportunity to learn and practice on an educational version of common electronic clinical systems before being required to use the production systems for actual patient care during their clinical experiences. This aspect is now expanded upon.

EDUCATIONAL ELECTRONIC MEDICAL RECORD

Having established that medical students should learn clinical informatics, including at least the basics of CDS, the electronic medical record (EMR) needs to be addressed. After medical students graduate and become residents, they will be expected to use the EMR to document patient care, place orders, review results and other data, and increasingly use dashboards and other analytics. At present, for most of these residents the extent of their training is a series of classes during residency orientation specific for their EMR that is intended to provide them with the minimum they need to function. However, the EMR is a complex system that has many ways to accomplish the same task, as well as sets of tools that can increase efficiency if used appropriately. With the recent changes in Centers for Medicare and Medicaid Services rules that allow physicians to verify medical student notes and use them for billing purposes, there will be an increasing demand for students during their clinical rotations to document directly into the patient chart.[38]

Given the need for medical students to learn how to appropriately and efficiently document in the EMR in addition to the educational needs of an informatics curriculum, the question becomes how to safely provide an environment for students to learn needed skills that can emulate the EMR without the risks of their working in a production environment. One suggestion is to develop and use an educational EMR (e-EMR) to provide this training and education. Other potential uses for an e-EMR is providing training in appropriate interactions with patients and computers during patient encounters, as well as appropriate professionalism in the use of communication tools and social media around patient care.[39,40]

An e-EMR is a simulated EMR environment that provides functionality similar to that of an actual EMR and contains a mix of patients specifically built for educational goals, as well as actual de-identified health data. The e-EMR should provide a student with a user experience close to that of an actual EMR. An e-EMR could be a separate "vendor-neutral" educational product or a specialized training environment of the academic health system's production EMR. Each option has its advantages and disadvantages. There are a myriad of potential uses for an e-EMR in undergraduate medical education.

Medical students need to learn clinical interviewing and accuracy of clinical documentation. One common educational activity in this area is the use of a Standardized Patient (SP) in simulating this common activity. Typically, students will interview patients while being observed and evaluated for their ability to obtain a history and their "bedside manner." The incorporation of an e-EMR into this simulation enables additional evaluation and guidance in how students interact with both a patient and technology simultaneously, how they document in the chart, and how they place orders.[41] Many of the existing electronic systems have the capability to document exactly where the student clicked and how long they spent in each area of the chart, thus enabling student evaluation and guidance toward the most efficient and effective use of the EMR.

Some of the more challenging patients that students and physicians need to care for are those with multiple chronic disease. Skills required include knowing how to effectively review a patient's chart, document accurately in the EMR, and use evidence-based tools to properly manage these complex patients. At OHSU, they have recreated this experience in simulated EHR Chronic Disease Management workshops. This tool has been offered to medical students during preclinical study and clerkships, as well as incoming internal medicine interns. Students review and update the simulated electronic chart of a patient with complex chronic disease, including placing orders for their patients, and are evaluated on their performance.[42]

By incorporating actual de-identified patient data into the e-EMR, students can learn about the wealth of data that is in actual patient records. The data are frequently not in a pristine form, and physicians need to learn how to work with real-world data. De-identified patient data also enable students to learn the principles of data analytics and the use of dashboards. By providing medical students and residents with knowledge of and access to data analytics tools, the next generation of physicians will be able to perform basic analytics themselves. Physicians will be able to obtain data analyses quickly and easily, supporting greater efficiency in patient care. In addition, this will free data analysts to focus on the more complex analyses for which their expertise is required. It is Geisinger's intent to roll out Epic's Slicer-Dicer analytics tool to its house staff during 2019. With appropriate training and education, it is hoped that residents will use Slicer-Dicer for their required quality and patient-safety projects in addition to patient care.

In CDS training, the e-EMR could be used in multiple different scenarios. Students can be exposed to CDS tools that are included in the e-EMR and accessed as part of their case-based or simulation classes. Examples of well-designed and poorly designed CDS interventions can be used to demonstrate and discuss the importance of these tools to the workflow of providers. Exercises whereby students design a CDS tool that is deployed to the e-EMR for analysis and evaluation will provide students with experience in CDS tool design and appreciation for the process of electronic tool development. At the graduate medical education level, pathology residents could focus their CDS development on tools surrounding the laboratory while residents from other training programs could work on tools important to their specialty of medicine. With cooperation across training programs within an institution, residents across specialties could work in teams to develop tools that incorporate multiple different clinical perspectives and help to build bridges between pathologists and their clinician partners.

Key features for using an e-EMR for undergraduate and graduate medical education in clinical informatics include the following.

1. *EMR training environment or educational product.* You have an option to use either a training environment of your EMR or a dedicated vendor-neutral educational EMR. Each has its advantages and disadvantages.
2. *Incorporate the e-EMR throughout education.* Although you can start with small pilot projects, the eventual goal is to use the e-EMR for all appropriate educational activities at multiple different educational levels.
3. *Engage and support your faculty.* One key to the effective use of the e-EMR is to engage your entire faculty and provide them with necessary training and support in the use of the e-EMR for education. This will require dedicated technical and educational support staff.
4. *Use both de-identified patient data and specific case scenarios.* De-identified actual patient data should be used as part of education in data science and analytics. Specific patient data will need to be built to support specific exercises throughout courses and simulations.
5. *Train students to use the EMR effectively.* Through the tracking features contained in these systems, students should be evaluated and guided in the use of tools that improve efficiency, support provider workflows, and are common throughout most commercial EMRs.
6. *CDS can be taught with e-EMR.* Students, residents, and physicians can all use CDS exercises in the e-EMR that enable them to recognize well-designed tools, assist them in understanding how to effectively participate in the development of CDS, and provide them with an appreciation for the potential of CDS tools in caring for patients.

PATHOLOGY RESIDENCY

Pathology has a long history of using informatics to support quality, safety, and the efficient operations of the laboratory.[15] This approach has resulted in informatics being so closely embedded into the practice of pathology that many pathologists do not recognize that they are also practicing informatics. Training in clinical informatics in general, and in pathology informatics and CDS specifically, is especially important for pathology residents. This fact has been recognized by the American Board of Pathology and the ACGME, where informatics has been incorporated into the Pathology

Residency Program Requirements and the Pathology Milestones, and informatics questions are asked on the pathology board examinations.[16,17,43]

In the Pathology Milestones, informatics is one of the systems-based practice subcompetencies. As residents progress through training, they are expected to move up the levels of the subcompetency by meeting the individual milestones at each level from 1 through 5. At Level 1, which is considered entry level for an incoming pathology resident, residents are expected to be familiar with basic computer hardware and software concepts. As they progress through residency, they would increase their knowledge regarding health and laboratory-specific informatics tools and then apply those tools in the practice of pathology in residency. The ACGME has established Level 4 as the target, not a requirement for graduation, and Level 5 as aspiration for residents but representing the expected informatics skills of pathologists after a few years in training.[43]

The challenge for Pathology Residency Program Directors and faculty is how to adequately educate and train pathology residents in the required aspects of clinical and pathology informatics. Pathology residency programs are already overloaded with rotations and educational sessions in the various disciplines of anatomic and clinical pathology, leaving very little time to include additional topics such as informatics and management. Residency faculty are not comfortable teaching informatics to residents. Despite their use of informatics day to day, few current faculty have any formal or informal training in pathology informatics. Also, most pathology residents, having little to no exposure to informatics during medical school and lacking informatics role models in residency, do not understand its importance and do not demand training.

There have been calls for informatics training in pathology residency and proposed models for learning objectives, outcomes, and possible structures for this training.[44-47] What became clear was that informatics education cannot be accomplished through a lecture series or a rotation in informatics during residency. Just as informatics is integrated into the daily practice of pathologists, training in informatics must be integrated into the entire residency curriculum. Furthermore, this education needs to be practical and include informatics exercises, focused on outcomes and what graduating residents can do instead of merely what they know.

In response to the growing recognition for informatics education in pathology residency and the challenges programs were facing in providing necessary instruction, the College of American Pathologists, Association of Pathology Chairs, and the Association for Pathology Informatics (API) collaborated on creating a pathology informatics curriculum for residents of pathology. The intent was to provide a program that any pathology residency program could implement, with or without a pathology informatician on faculty.

A group of 20 pathology informaticians and educators, with an eye toward the Pathology ACGME Milestones and the new subspecialty examination in clinical informatics, identified 38 essential pathology informatics competencies and organized them into the 4 levels of the PIER. Along with outcome statements for each of the competencies is included the rationale and the content for the competency, references and other resources, and practical exercises that demonstrate knowledge of and/or experience with the competency.[18]

Since the initial release in 2014, PIER has continued to advance. As of September 2018, PIER is currently in Release Version 3, where the content has been reviewed and updated in a rapidly evolving field. Additional content has been added, including a mapping between the PIER Essentials to recorded presentations from API's informatics boot camps and conference presentations.[48] Penetration of the PIER curriculum throughout pathology residency programs continues to struggle because of the similar issues of lack of time within training to add informatics and the lack of dedicated and trained informatics faculty.[49]

Within PIER, decision support is included as a part of the PIER Essentials Level 4 topic of Orders & Results Management. The practical exercises include activities that can be incorporated into one or more rotation involving the ordering and display of laboratory tests. One of the program recommendations is to create a teaching file of examples or problems involving computerized provider order entry for laboratory tests.[50] To build on PIER, programs might consider incorporating additional exercises, such as the medical student decision support activity described by the MUSC.[37] Pathology residents can actively participate in the development, deployment, and analysis of CDS tools involving laboratory ordering, reflex ordering, or results interpretation.

Pathology is not the only specialty struggling with the issue of incorporating informatics education into residency programs. The challenges of incorporating informatics training into residency programs is common across specialties and include already overloaded residency curricula and lack of adequately trained faculty within each program. One possible path forward is to have residency programs within an institution combine resources to offer this training cooperatively. Much of the content could be provided online, and discussion groups could be offered both intraresidency and across multiple residencies as needed. Practical exercises, such as CDS tool development, would best be offered to multispecialty teams of residents to solve together.

Another alternative is to use some common educational activities across pathology residency programs at different academic institutions to provide required informatics training. This content can be provided commercially, such as with the American Society for Clinical Pathology's and Association for Pathology Informatics' University of Pathology Informatics.[51] Informatics content can also be developed by the programs themselves and shared cooperatively across academic institutions, as has been successfully accomplished within the informatics community. The Clinical Informatics Fellowship Programs offer a monthly Virtual Case Conference (VCC) in which informatics concepts are presented through case-based scenarios on a rotating basis by different fellowship programs. The goal of the VCC is to present topics that fellows may not be exposed to during their training, such as a security breach and how to respond. The pathology informatics community initiated a series of fellow retreats that also used case-based scenarios to teach fellows across different training programs.[52] This approach has been duplicated in the clinical informatics community as an annual retreat.

The key features for providing appropriate training in decision support and informatics for pathology residents include the following.

1. *An informatics foundation is necessary.* Training pathology residents in CDS tools needs to be part of a sufficiently broad education in clinical and pathology informatics. This must be part of every residency regardless of the extent of informatics training students may have had in medical school.
2. *CDS is not just about placing orders.* CDS can help providers to order the appropriate test for the right patient at the right time; but CDS can also assist with complex reflex testing and in helping providers and patients understand laboratory results and possible next steps forward.
3. *Informatics is more than a lecture or rotation.* Informatics is inseparable from the practice of pathology. By extension, informatics education must be integrated

into the curriculum and through all pathology residency rotations as appropriate and relevant.

4. *Informatics training is hands-on.* Although informatics knowledge is important, residents will best learn informatics skills through practice in both simulated exercises and actual informatics activities within the laboratory.

5. *Look at things through a clinician's eyes.* Although knowledge of the technical aspects of CDS is important, one must not forget that informatics is a team sport and that the perspective of clinicians using CDS tools is critical. Collaboration with other residency programs to hold joint educational activities on CDS and informatics is essential.

6. *Collaborate with other training programs.* Reach out and collaborate with other residency programs in your institution or other pathology residency programs at other academic medical centers to provide necessary education in informatics and CDS. Everyone is looking to provide this education while struggling to find the required resources.

CLINICAL INFORMATICS AND PATHOLOGY INFORMATICS FELLOWSHIPS

Clinical informatics fellowships are a relatively recent development in medical education. The ACGME first promulgated the clinical informatics program requirements and accredited the first 4 fellowship programs in 2014. One of the 4 initially accredited fellowship programs is based in pathology.[53] In September 2018, among the 32 ACGME-accredited fellowship programs in clinical informatics, 7 are based in pathology departments, more than any other specialty aside from internal medicine.[54]

The National Board of Medical Specialties officially recognized clinical informatics as a subspecialty of medicine in 2011. The 2 sponsoring boards are the American Board of Pathology (ABPath) and the American Board of Preventive Medicine (ABPM). Since the initiation of board examinations in 2013, the ABPath has offered the clinical informatics board examination for all pathologists while the ABPM administers the examination for all other medical specialties.

It is not a surprise that pathology is strongly represented in clinical informatics. For many years before board certification and ACGME fellowships, there have been a small number of pathology informatics fellowship programs offered. First conceived as an apprentice-like experience, pathology informatics grew into a formal unaccredited fellowship program with a well-defined curriculum, program requirements, different tracks, and national fellow retreats.[29,52,55,56]

Instruction and extensive practical experiences involving CDS is a standard feature among both pathology informatics and clinical informatics fellowships.[28,29] These fellows represent an invaluable educational resource to assist in educating medical students and residents in CDS as well as the broader field of informatics. In addition, the educational activities within the fellowships can be extended to provide the same training to pathology residents. Residents can be included in educational sessions on CDS, and can be partnered with informatics fellows working on decision support projects.

There has been significant discussion around the topic of combined or blended fellowships. The concept is to combine or blend a clinical informatics fellowship with a subspecialty fellowship to provide synergy in training across the 2 subspecialty disciplines. It is thought that a pathologist simultaneously training in a path subspecialty and informatics will integrate the knowledge of both subspecialties, focus them together, and strengthen the overall training. Interest in different tracks for informatics training originated in the pathology community.[56] The American Board of Pathology formally approved combining the 2-year clinical informatics fellowship with a 1-year pathology subspecialty fellowship into a single 2-year program that would allow pathologists to qualify for both board examinations.[57]

The key features for fellowships in clinical and pathology informatics' relationship to training pathologists in CDS include the following.

1. *Leverage other informatics educational programs.* There is significant overlap in informatics and CDS educational goals and outcomes for medical students, residents, and fellows. Use existing educational resources when available or combine efforts with similar initiatives to achieve common goals.
2. *Fellows are an invaluable resource.* Do not forget to reach out to your institution's clinical or pathology informatics fellowship program to engage fellows in educational activities and projects with residents.
3. *Consider the advantages of blended fellowships.* A fellowship that combines and blends a pathology subspecialty and clinical/pathology informatics is an excellent way to educate pathologists in both fields and enhances their knowledge and use of tools such as CDS as part of their practice.

CONTINUING MEDICAL EDUCATION

At present, appropriate informatics and CDS training for practicing physicians in general and pathologists specifically is mostly overlooked. Why are we surprised when clinicians ignore or fight against the deployment of CDS tools when the overwhelming majority of them have had no significant education in this area? With appropriate education and support, most physicians will have a better understanding of data, the need for appropriate data entry by clinicians into the EMR, and how that data can be used to improve patient care, leading to a greater acceptance of CDS tools, better compliance with well-designed CDS interventions, and positive feedback on how to improve poorly designed CDS interventions. Similarly, pathologists and laboratorians who have little to no knowledge of the potential for CDS tools should not be expected to invest their limited time in helping to develop these tools. Although decision support has not yet affected the practice of pathologists directly, tools to advise pathologists on appropriate follow-up or reflex testing are being developed. The emergence of computational pathology will require significant retraining of existing pathologists and laboratorians in the principles of informatics and CDS.[58]

Given the similarities in the informatics curriculum at multiple educational levels, content that has been developed to educate and train our medical students, residents, and fellows can be used to provide informatics education at the continuing medical education (CME) level. Practicing pathologists could make use of online content that has already been developed for informatics education. Practical exercises in CDS tool development and optimization could be offered to physicians at all levels jointly. Partnering medical students, residents, and physicians in teams to work together on these exercises will allow each level of student to share their perspective. Practicing physicians and pathologists have a wealth of clinical experience as well as frustrations and successes in using electronic tools, including CDS, as part of their medical practice. Students and residents bring their lifelong knowledge and experiences of being the first generation raised as consumers of data and using electronic tools from childhood. Informatics fellows can function as the facilitators of these practical sessions and act as a bridge between the students/residents and physicians/pathologists.

The key points to remember for informatics and CDS education at the practicing pathologist level are as follows.

1. *Don't forget to educate at all levels.* Physicians already in practice lack significant training in informatics and require appropriate CME. This lack of informatics knowledge at the faculty level has had a negative impact on our ability to train medical students and residents.
2. *Use already existing content where relevant.* There is no need to reinvent the wheel for informatics CME. Use already existing content when available, both inside and outside your institution, to provide necessary knowledge.
3. *Facilitate multidisciplinary and multilevel training.* With informatics and CDS practical exercises, leverage the strength of combined training. Each professional brings his or her unique perspective and experiences to these exercises.

REFERENCES

1. Procop GW, Yerian LM, Wyllie R, et al. Duplicate laboratory test reduction using a clinical decision support tool. Am J Clin Pathol 2014;141:718–23.
2. Bellodi E, Vagnoni E, Bonvento B, et al. Economic and organizational impact of a clinical decision support system on laboratory test ordering. BMC Med Inform Decis Mak 2017;17:179.
3. Eaton KP, Chida N, Apfel A, et al. Impact of nonintrusive clinical decision support systems on laboratory test utilization in a large academic center. J Eval Clin Pract 2018;24:474–9.
4. Sikaris K. Enhancing the clinical value of medical laboratory testing. Clin Biochem Rev 2017;38:107–14.
5. Baron JM, Dighe AS. The role of informatics and decision support in utilization management. Clin Chim Acta 2014;427:196–201.
6. Kopanitsa G, Semenov I. Patient facing decision support systems for interpretation of laboratory test results. BMC Med Inform Decis Mak 2018;16:68.
7. Yeh ML, Chang YJ, Wang PY, et al. Physicians' responses to computerized drug-drug interaction alerts for outpatients. Comput Methods Programs Biomed 2013; 111:17–25.
8. Carli D, Fahrni G, Bonnabry P, et al. Quality of decision support in computerized provider order entry: systematic literature review. JMIR Med Inform 2018;6:e3.
9. Delvaux N, Thienen KV, Heselmans A, et al. The effects of computerized clinical decision support systems on laboratory test ordering: a systematic review. Arch Pathol Lab Med 2017;141:585–95.
10. Rubenstein M, Hirsch R, Bandyopadhyay K, et al. Effectiveness of practices to support appropriate laboratory test utilization. Am J Clin Pathol 2018;149: 197–221.
11. Bates DW, Kuperman GJ, Wang S, et al. Ten commandments for effective clinical decision support: making the practice of evidence-based medicine a reality. J Am Med Inform Assoc 2003;10:523–30.
12. Baron JM, Lewandrowski KB, Kamis IK, et al. A novel strategy for evaluating the effects of an electronic test ordering alert message: optimizing cardiac marker usage. J Pathol Inform 2012;3:3.
13. Rudolf JW, Dighe AS, Coley CM, et al. Analysis of daily laboratory orders at a large urban academic center: a multifaceted approach to changing test ordering patterns. Am J Clin Pathol 2017;148:128–35.
14. Shirts BH, Jackson BR, Baird GS, et al. Clinical laboratory analytics: challenges and promise for an emerging discipline. J Pathol Inform 2015;6:9.
15. Park S, Parwani AV, Aller RD, et al. The history of pathology informatics: a global perspective. J Pathol Inform 2013;4:7.

16. Accreditation Council for Graduate Medical Education. ACGME program requirements for graduate medical education in anatomic pathology and clinical pathology 2018. Available at: https://acgme.org/Portals/0/PFAssets/ProgramRequirements/300PathologyCore2018.pdf?ver=2018-02-19-085552-553. Accessed September, 2018.

17. American Board of Pathology. Clinical pathology exam blueprint 2018. Available at: http://abpath.org/index.php/taking-an-examination/primary-certificate-requirements. Accessed September, 2018.

18. Henricks WH, Karcher DS, Harrison JH Jr, et al. Pathology informatics essentials for residents: a flexible informatics curriculum linked to accreditation council for graduate medical education milestones. J Pathol Inform 2016;7:27.

19. Flexner A. Medical education in the United States and Canada. Washington, DC: Science and Health Publications, Inc.; 1910.

20. Pershing S, Fuchs VR. Restructuring medical education to meet current and future health care needs. Acad Med 2013;88:1798–801.

21. Beaudoin DE, Richardson SJ, Sheng X, et al. Medical students' perspectives on biomedical informatics learning objectives. Int J Med Educ 2013;4:1–8.

22. Banerjee R, George P, Priebe C, et al. Medical student awareness of and interest in clinical informatics. J Am Med Inform Assoc 2015;22:e42–7.

23. The Informatics Panel and the Population Health Perspective Panel. Contemporary issues in medicine—medical informatics and population health: report ii of the medical school objectives project. Acad Med 1999;74:130–41.

24. Gonzalo JD, Dekhtyar M, Starr SR, et al. Health systems science curricula in undergraduate medical education: identifying and defining a potential curricular framework. Acad Med 2017;92:123–31.

25. Liaison Committee on Medical Education. Medical education questionnaire part II. Chicago: American Medical Association; 2008.

26. Richardson JE, Bouquin DR, Tmanova LL, et al. Information and informatics literacies of first-year medical students. J Med Libr Assoc 2015;103:198–202.

27. Badgett RG, Paukert JL, Levy LS. Teaching clinical informatics to third-year medical students: negative results from two controlled trials. BMC Med Educ 2001;1:3.

28. Gardner RM, Overhage JM, Steen EB, et al. Core content for the subspecialty of clinical informatics. J AM Med Inform Assoc 2009;16:153–7.

29. McClintock DS, Levy BP, Lane WJ, et al. A core curriculum for clinical fellowship training in pathology informatics. J Pathol Inform 2012;3:31.

30. International Medical Informatics Association. Recommendations of the International Medical Informatics Association (IMIA) on education in health and medical informatics. Methods Inf Med 2000;39:267–77.

31. Mantas J, Ammenwerth E, Demiris G, et al. Recommendations of the International Medical Informatics Association (IMIA) on education in health and medical informatics: first revision. Methods Inf Med 2010;49:105–20.

32. Winter A, Hilgers R, Hofestadt R, et al. More than four decades of medical informatics education for medical students in Germany. Methods Inf Med 2013;52:181–3.

33. Berber ES, Boulware DW. Medical informatics for medical students: not just because it's there. Med Educ Online 1996;1. https://doi.org/10.3402/meo.v1i.4283.

34. McGowan J, Raszka W, Light J, et al. A vertical curriculum to teach the knowledge, skills, and attitudes of medical informatics. Proc AMIA Symp 1998;457–61.

35. Silverman H, Cohen T, Fridsma D. The evolution of a novel biomedical informatics curriculum for medical students. Acad Med 2012;87:84–90.

36. Hersh WR, Gorman PN, Biagioli FE, et al. Beyond information retrieval and electronic health record use: competencies in clinical informatics for medical education. Adv Med Educ Pract 2014;5:205–12.

37. Crabtree EA, Brennan E, Davis A, et al. Connecting education to quality: engaging medical students in the development of evidence-based clinical decision support tools. Acad Med 2017;92:83–6.

38. Centers for Medicare and Medicaid Services. Guidelines for teaching physicians, interns, and residents (ICN 006347) 2018. Available at: https://www.cms.gov/Outreach-and-Education/Medicare-Learning-Network-MLN/MLNProducts/Downloads/Teaching-Physicians-Fact-Sheet-ICN006437.pdf. Accessed September, 2018.

39. Mostaghimi A, Olszewski AE, Bell SK, et al. Erosion of digital professionalism during medical students' core clinical clerkships. JMIR Med Educ 2017;3:e9.

40. Wald HS, George P, Reis SP, et al. Electronic heath record training in undergraduate medical education: bridging theory to practice with curricula for empowering patient-a and relationship-centered care in the computerized setting. Acad Med 2014;89:380–6.

41. Biagioli FE, Elliot DL, Palmer RT, et al. The electronic health record objective structured clinical examination: assessing student competency in patient interactions while using the electronic health record. Acad Med 2017;92:87–91.

42. Hersch W, Biagioli F, Scholl G, et al. From competencies to competence: model, approach, and lessons learned from implementing a clinical informatics curriculum for medical students. In: Shachak A, Borycki EM, Reis SP, editors. Health professionals' education in the age of clinical information systems, mobile computing and social networks. London: Elsevier; 2017. p. 269–87.

43. Accreditation Council for Graduate Medical Education and The American Board of Pathology. The pathology milestone project 2015. Available at: https://acgme.org/Portals/0/PDFs/Milestones/PathologyMilestones.pdf?ver=2017-10-09-125324-230. Accessed September, 2018.

44. Henricks WH, Healy JC. Informatics training in pathology residency programs. Am J Clin Pathol 2002;118:172–8.

45. Henricks WH, Boyer PJ, Harrison JH, et al. Informatics training in pathology residency programs: proposed learning objectives and skill sets for the new millennium. Arch Pathol Lab Med 2003;127:1009–18.

46. Rao LKF, Gilbertson JR. Longitudinal engagement of pathology residents: a proposed approach for informatics training. Am J Clin Pathol 2014;142:748–54.

47. Sinard JH, Powell SZ, Karcher DS. Pathology training in informatics: evolving to meet a growing need. Arch Pathol Lab Med 2014;138:505–11.

48. Association for Pathology Chairs. Pathology informatics essentials for residents 2018. Available at: https://apc.memberclicks.net/index.php?option=com_content&view=article&id=152:pier&catid=20:site-content&Itemid=156. Accessed September, 2018.

49. Anderson SR. Informatics Working Group and PIER Update. Presented at Association for Pathology Chairs Annual Meeting. San Diego, July 16, 2018. Available at: https://s3.amazonaws.com/v3-app_crowdc/assets/3/3b/3b0ddbf40ac6fb12/1115_S_Anderson_071618.original.1533070929.pdf?1533070933. Accessed September, 2018.

50. Association for Pathology Chairs, Association for Pathology Informatics, College of American Pathologists. Pathology Informatics essentials for residents: PIER

resource toolkit 2018. Available at: https://apc.memberclicks.net/assets/docs/pier/PIER%20Toolkit%20R3.pdf. Accessed September, 2018.

51. American Society for Clinical Pathology and Association for Pathology Informatics, University of Pathology Informatics. 2018. Available at: https://www.ascp.org/content/learning/certificate-programs. Accessed September, 2018.

52. Lee RE, McCintock DS, Balis UJ, et al. Pathology informatics fellowship retreats: the use of interactive scenarios and case studies as pathology informatics teaching tools. J Pathol Inform 2012;3:41.

53. Longhurst CA, Pageler NM, Palma JP, et al. Early experiences of accredited clinical informatics fellowships. J Am Med Inform Assoc 2016;23:829–34.

54. Accreditation Council for Graduate Medical Education (ACGME)—Public. 2018. Available at: https://apps.acgme.org/ads/Public. Accessed September, 2018.

55. Gilbertson JR, McClintock DS, Lee RE, et al. Clinical fellowship training in pathology informatics: a program description. J Pathol Inform 2012;3:11.

56. Levy BP, McClintock DS, Lee RE, et al. Different tracks for pathology informatics fellowship training: experiences of and input from trainees in a large multisite fellowship program. J Pathol Inform 2012;3:30.

57. American Board of Pathology. Clinical informatics requirements for certification 2018. Available at: http://www.abpath.org/index.php/to-become-certified/requirements-for-certification?id=40. Accessed September, 2018.

58. Louis DN, Feldman M, Carter AB, et al. Computational pathology: a path ahead. Arch Pathol Lab Med 2016;140:41–50.

Machine Learning and Other Emerging Decision Support Tools

Jason M. Baron, MD*, Danielle E. Kurant, MD,
Anand S. Dighe, MD, PhD

KEYWORDS

- Machine learning • Clinical decision support • Artificial intelligence
- Knowledge discovery • Computational pathology

KEY POINTS

- Artificial intelligence offers the potential to develop enhanced decision support that can support a wide range of clinical decisions with a high degree of patient specificity.
- The foundation of many emerging decision support techniques is machine leaning-based knowledge discovery, in which existing patient medical records are "mined" for new insights.
- Technical, administrative, and education challenges are widespread, but solutions to some of these may be on the horizon.

LIMITATIONS OF TRADITIONAL APPROACHES TO CLINICAL DECISION SUPPORT

Laboratory clinical decision support (CDS) has traditionally focused on helping clinicians apply medical knowledge derived from traditional knowledge sources to care for patients. For example, test ordering alert messages may be deployed within computerized provider order entry systems during the test ordering process to provide just-in-time information about the appropriate indications for testing.[1–6] Examples of traditional types of CDS are detailed in other articles within this issue.

Although traditional CDS provides an invaluable toolset in optimizing test selection and test result interpretation, traditional CDS suffers from certain key limitations (**Fig. 1**). In particular, traditional systems often lack optimal patient specificity while providing support for only a small percentage of the various laboratory-diagnostic

Disclosure Statement: In addition to his academic role, Dr J.M. Baron works part-time as a computational pathologist for Roche Diagnostics. The other authors have nothing to disclose.
Department of Pathology, Massachusetts General Hospital, Harvard Medical School, 55 Fruit Street, Boston, MA 02214, USA
* Corresponding author. Massachusetts General Hospital, Ruth Sleeper Hall Rm 180A, 55 Fruit Street, Boston, MA 02114.
E-mail address: jmbaron@partners.org

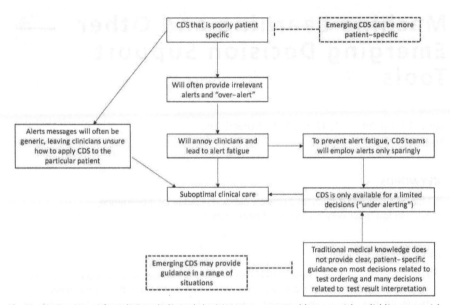

Fig. 1. Limitations of traditional clinical decision support. Red boxes with solid lines provide a schematic of some of the limitations of traditional clinical decision support (CDS). The green boxes with dashed lines show how emerging technologies may offer new opportunities to enhance CDS.

decisions that a clinician must make. For example, many test ordering alert messages are built to "pop-up" rather indiscriminately every time a physician attempts to order a test. An example of this would be an alert that fires every time a physician attempts to order a creatine kinase MB band test advising that this is not the best test to evaluate myocardial infarction.[7] Alternatively, alerts may use rather rudimentary rules to determine when to fire, in turn leading to frequent over- or under-alerting; for example, a flag that alerts clinicians to the possibility of acute kidney injury anytime a patient experiences a substantial increase in plasma creatinine may falsely alert on dialysis patients who commonly experience wide fluctuations in creatinine before and after dialysis treatment.[8]

Indiscriminate alerting, particularly when frequent, will typically lead to clinician annoyance and "alert fatigue" in which clinicians ignore alerts.[1,3] When working with alerts that are not optimally patient specific, the usual approach to avoiding alert fatigue is to limit the number of alerts used. However, this under-alerting also has consequences as it leaves most clinical decisions unsupported. Given these limitations of traditional CDS, decision support strategies that are highly patient-specific or that provide information that the clinician would not have otherwise known may yield immense clinical value, and, indeed, these next-generation decision support strategies are beginning to emerge. The often-mentioned field of "computational pathology" aims in large part to advance the development and implementation of these evolving types of CDS by mining new insights from patient data within electronic health record (EHR) systems and applying this knowledge in the form of patient-specific CDS.[9–11]

THREE COMPONENTS OF AN EMERGING CLINICAL DECISION SUPPORT STRATEGY

As illustrated in **Fig. 2**, this article divides the requirements for computational pathology and patient-specific emerging CDS into 3 components: knowledge discovery,

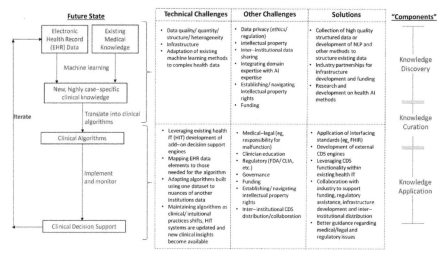

Fig. 2. A 3-component model of an emerging CDS strategy, providing a framework for an emerging CDS strategy that first mines existing health records to provide new clinical insights, then translates these finding into clinical algorithms, and finally implements the clinical algorithms as a CDS. For each step, various challenges and considerations are described.

knowledge curation, and knowledge application. Whereas this division into 3 components is admittedly an oversimplification, and successful approaches to patient-specific CDS might not neatly break apart into these 3 components, the authors nonetheless think that this framework is useful. Major advances in any of these 3 components would go a long way toward advancing computational pathology as a whole.

Knowledge discovery (see **Fig. 2**) involves generating new clinical knowledge by mining "real world data" (RWD) contained within EHRs. Although subsequent sections will discuss data mining in greater detail, it is important to first consider a more fundamental question: Why do we need to derive new knowledge from RWD and why can we not just base all CDS on traditional sources of knowledge such as clinical trials, retrospective studies, expert opinion, and consensus guidelines? The short answer is that we can and should incorporate existing knowledge, but existing knowledge alone is not enough. Traditional clinical knowledge can be very informative when it is available and directly relevant to a given clinical decision, and high-quality randomized controlled trials contribute invaluable and irreplaceable knowledge to our medical corpus; however, existing clinical knowledge will fail to directly address most clinical decisions. For example, most laboratory test ordering decisions cannot be supported by an authoritative expert opinion, let alone a high-quality clinical trial. Likewise, even when trials do exist, patients at hand may not match exactly the inclusion/exclusion criteria of the trial, leaving doubt as to whether the results from the trial are applicable. Perhaps most importantly, traditional medical knowledge will often fail to achieve the desired patient specificity. For example, we may know from a clinical trial that 25% of patients with disorder X respond to therapy Y. "But how do I know whether my patient will be one of the non-responders and should I consider therapy Z instead?" Simply mining RWD data will not alone provide an answer to every clinical question, but it certainly has potential to provide new insights and greater patient specificity.

Similarly, simply discovering new clinical knowledge is also insufficient; clinical knowledge does little good if not disseminated in a form that can be applied to clinical decision-making. In addition to publication, findings from RWD can often be translated directly into "clinical algorithms" (knowledge curation phase of **Fig. 2**). Using the 3-component framework described above, clinical algorithms represent the embodiment of clinical knowledge in a form that applies patient information as inputs and generates one or more elements of diagnostic, prognostic, or prescriptive information as an output.

MACHINE LEARNING: THE WORKHORSE OF KNOWLEDGE DISCOVERY

Although a comprehensive review of machine learning is outside the scope of this article, numerous other resources provide basic and in-depth discussions and tutorials on this topic.[12] The purpose of this section is to provide a high-level conceptual overview; the discussion here is intended to provide intuition and is not intended to be a computationally rigorous description.

The arguably most important type of machine learning for computational pathology, *supervised* machine learning, trains a model to predict an outcome of interest ("target variable" or "dependent variable") based on some other information within the dataset ("predictors" or "features"). A schematic showing the process of developing a supervised machine-learning model is shown in **Fig. 3**. As shown, supervised machine-learning algorithms are always trained on a set of *labeled* training data with labels representing the "ground truth" (gold standard values) for the outcome of interest. The data used to train, test, and apply supervised machine learning often takes the form of a 2D table with rows (by convention) representing cases (eg, patients) and columns representing feature and outcome variables (see **Fig. 3**). Often, one of the first steps in a machine-learning problem is to define the outcome of interest and select the data elements that will be used to predict this outcome. The process of selecting predictors is called "feature selection" and is sometimes in part empiric.

There are hundreds if not thousands of different types of machine-learning models, including simple regression (eg, linear regression/logistic regression), tree-based methods (decision trees and random forests), support vector machines and neural networks. The type of model determines the general form (eg, shape) that the predictive algorithm will take and the approach that will be used to train (eg, fit) this general form to the training data. Model selection is an important step and is often largely empiric, but data science and domain expertise can be helpful. Often multiple types are tested and sometimes combined into the final prediction algorithm. Of note, when discussing machine learning, one term that can be confusing is "algorithm"; the term algorithm can be used to describe the type of model (eg, a neural network) or the final output (eg, a diagnostic algorithm that is based on a neural network). This review uses the terms "type of model" and "prediction algorithm" to improve clarity.

Although the type of model defines the general form, model "training" defines the specific relationships between the predictors and the outcomes. In most cases, model training involves, in large part, optimizing the values of mathematical *parameters* that determine the predictions that the trained prediction model will calculate for a given set of input predictors. Parameters will sometimes be set to make the prediction algorithm's predicted outcomes best match the ground truth labels on the training data. For example, with least mean squares regression, which can be used as a machine-learning algorithm in addition to its more widely known statistical application, the parameters are the coefficients and these are set to minimize the squared residuals. In more sophisticated machine-learning frameworks, parameters are typically optimized to minimize the value of a "cost function" that may consider additional factors related to the generalizability of the model.

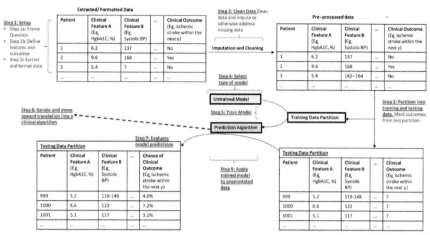

Fig. 3. Schematic of supervised machine learning. Shown is a schematic of a typical framework for using machine learning in clinical knowledge discovery. Step 1 involves framing the problem and extracting the data. Key considerations in this step include deciding which features (predictors) to use in the model and how to define and extract the specific features and outcomes. Significant domain expertise is often needed. Step 2 involves data cleaning and imputation of missing data. Data cleaning may involve removal of anomalous or inconsistent data and applying groupers to categorize similar data elements together. Missing data can be imputed by inferring the most likely values or range for a missing data element based on the data that are available. The cleaned data are then often partitioned into training and testing datasets (step 3); if the test partition is derived after cleaning and imputation, the researchers must take care to ensure that outcome information from the original dataset does not leak into the testing partition. Step 3 can be omitted or modified if an independently derived dataset is to be used for testing. The type of model must be selected (step 4) and trained (step 5). Training may involve cross-validation to fit hyperparameters ("tuning") and to provide a preliminary assessment of test data performance. The trained model can then be applied to the test partition or an independent set of test data (step 6) and predicted outcomes can be compared with ground truth values, which would generally have been collected but masked to assess model performance (step 7). This process is often iterative (step 8). In practice, there is often overlap between various steps (eg, training can inform feature selection). It should also be noted that, in many problems, most of the effort required for steps 1 through 7 is invested into step 1 and sometimes to a lesser extent step 2.

After a model is trained, it is important to test the model on an independent set of test data not used in the training. This is to ensure that model performance is generalizable and is not overfit as described below.

OVERFITTING AND TRAINING DATA NEEDS

An often-asked question in the context of machine-learning projects is, "How much data do I need?" The answer is that it depends on model complexity. Whereas the formal mathematics of model complexity are described in many other sources and are outside the scope of this article, in general, models are *more complex* if they include a greater number of predictors and/or parameters and allow for more complex relationships between predictors and outcomes. More complex models will require a larger number of cases in the training data to be properly fit. An intuitive way of thinking about this is that more parameters will provide a model more options to get from the predictors to the outcome, and thus more cases will be needed to determine which of these options is most correct. If too few cases are used to train a complex model, it will tend to *overfit*. An overfit model will identify happenstantial nuances of the training data that by chance associate with the various outcomes but do not represent real relationships between features and outcomes. For example, by way of analogy, a Boston Red Sox fan might compare her own *personal* daily activities to whether the Sox win; given enough factors relative to the number of games examined, she might find that the Sox win when she has orange juice with breakfast and wears black shoes. This would almost certainly represent an overfit model. An overfit model will tend to perform much better on the training data than on an independent set of test data because the happenstantial nuances the model fit to in the training data will usually not be present in an independent set of test data. For example, the Red Sox fan's model involving orange juice and shoe color will be unlikely to generalize to the following season. Overfitting is measured based on the difference between training and testing data performance. Testing data performance, as opposed to training data performance, is what really matters when evaluating the potential utility of a predictive algorithm.

When planning a machine-learning project, a key is that the model complexity must be appropriate for the amount of training data available. If limited data are available, a less complex model may be considered. However, because a simplistic model may be insufficient to meet performance goals, a large quantity of data may be needed for certain problems. Because a goal of computational pathology is to achieve a high degree of patient specificity, complex models and large datasets are likely to be needed in many cases. This would likely be best achieved through inter-institutional data sharing, but this has its own challenges, as noted below.

CHALLENGES AND SOLUTIONS IN KNOWLEDGE DISCOVERY

Although many of the machine-learning methods needed for knowledge discovery are readily available, both technical and administrative challenges remain. Key technical challenges relate to limitations of data quality, quantity, and structure. Administrative challenges relate to gaining access to needed data in light of regulatory and legal requirements and business strategy considerations.

Need for Better Mechanisms to Share Data

As alluded to previously, the types of models that will be most useful in advancing computational pathology may be complex and incorporate a large number of features, and thus require a large set of cases for training. Particularly in the setting of rare diagnoses and clinical conditions, any single institution is unlikely to alone have a sufficient number of cases. Moreover, many talented data scientists and data science resources reside in industry or non-clinical academic settings and outside the types of large health systems likely to have internal access to substantial clinical data. Thus, there are often mismatches between data science resources and data. To fully leverage available data to the benefit of patients, the field will need to overcome barriers to data sharing and inter-institutional data pooling.

Administrative Challenges

Arguably, the most significant barriers to data sharing and the more expeditious use of RWD in the development of new clinical knowledge are administrative. In particular, in the authors' experience, many health care systems are reluctant to share data externally for several reasons. Foremost, institutions are appropriately concerned about patient privacy and security. Although risks to patient privacy can be partially miti-gated through proper de-identification, when working with large datasets, there is sometimes a risk that data, even when de-identified to the HIPAA standard, can be re-identified by linking the data to other available data sources.[13] Moreover, thorough de-identification can be quite difficult in many settings; for example, narrative notes may inadvertently provide identifying clues such as that the patient has a certain job title. Likewise, identifiers such as dates may be needed in building models. Although some relevant identifiers can be obscured, others cannot. For example, dates can usually be shifted to convey relative as opposed to absolute time, but certain social variables may be difficult to obscure without losing information. Extracting and de-identifying data can itself be a significant effort; some systems may have limited re-sources for doing this internally.

Even with de-identified data, health systems may be justifiably concerned about losing control of data once sent to third parties. Although sharers of data will generally require the receiving party to sign a data use agreement governing terms of data use and potentially stipulating that data must be deleted by the receiving party at the conclusion of the specified project, breaches of such agreements may be difficult for the data sharer to detect. Data sharers may also be concerned about security breaches within the receiving institution. Health systems may retain control of data and mitigate the risk of unauthorized data use by insisting that third parties access the data only on servers within the sharing health system's firewall; however, this will require the health system to supply suitable computing resources internally, which might not always be feasible. Issues of patient consent and compliance with regulation must also be considered. The legal and ethical issues related to who owns and who can use data for which purposes are outside the authors' area of expertise and outside the scope of this article; however, of course, these are substantial issues. (Do patients own their data? Do hospitals?)[14] Finally, health systems are increasingly recognizing the potential economic value of their health care data and would understandably like to use their data resources to provide a revenue stream or obtain intellectual prop-erty rights in products derived from their data. These financial considerations may complicate or hinder the formation of certain data sharing arrangements.

Data Quality and Structure

Data quality will often limit the use of data in secondary analyses and algorithm training. Most types of machine-learning models rely on predictors and outcomes that are structured. However, real clinical data elements may exist in narrative notes and other outcomes that cannot be directly entered into machine-learning algorithms. Various pre-processing steps such as using natural language processing can help, but these technologies have their limits and may introduce an unacceptable amount of noise or error. Furthermore, even when data are structured, a substantial amount of work may be required to identify the underlying meaning of various data elements and to properly extract the dataset. These data extraction and normalization chal-lenges will be compounded when pooling data across multiple sources, such as from different institutions. Mapping data to standards (eg, SNOMED, LOINC) might help, but will not entirely solve this challenge.[15-18]

Perhaps the biggest challenges to analyzing clinical data are data accuracy, completeness, and heterogeneity. RWD will never include every data element that might be potentially be useful for a model. For example, no patient will have every possible laboratory test. Likewise, certain types of clinical data (eg, billing codes) are notoriously inaccurate. Finally, data heterogeneity is a major challenge. Most machine-learning models will work best (or will only work) with complete datasets that contain a value for every predictor; however, constructing these types of datasets directly is often impossible and manual curation may be required. For example, in an inter-institutional dataset, patients may have vitamin D measured by immunoassay or by mass-spectroscopy, but not both. Thus, domain expertise, empiric evaluation, or a combination of the two, may be needed to determine whether vitamin D, by each method, can be treated interchangeably in the model. Similarly, if a data scientist wishes to use results for 30 different laboratory tests in a model, few patients will have results for all 30. A solution might be to remove features that are missing in a large fraction of patients. Remaining features that are only missing in a minor fraction of patients can then be imputed for those patients in whom they are missing. Imputation methods are commonly used and imputation has been described previously.[19–24] The missing data problem becomes particularly significant when considering temporally based models.[20] For example, if time is divided with sufficient granularity (eg, to the minute) most patients will not have most observations (eg, test results) recorded at most time points. Various methods are available to model time series data including taking time "windows" and then featurizing time (eg, using the mean, minimum, and maximum value for a test in a patient each day if there are multiple repeat tests), but this can discard important information concerning temporal trends and inter-relationships between various observations over time. The authors of this article developed and proposed a new method, "3D-MICE," to impute missing results over time, thus potentially enabling secondary predictive models to incorporate laboratory test results at any arbitrary time point as predictors.[20] The specific utility of 3D-MICE in addressing the challenge of modeling time series-based data for use in predictive models remains to be fully established, but the authors would encourage interested researchers to consider whether 3D-MICE might provide a useful tool in their own analyses.

TRANSLATING KNOWLEDGE INTO CLINICAL ALGORITHMS
General Considerations

A trained machine-learning model is not itself a "clinical algorithm" ready for implementation. Additional details must be considered and worked out including what will "trigger" the model to run, what the output will be, how the output will be communicated to end users (eg, clinicians), and how the end users should be directed to act on the output. For example, a multiple analyte "synthetic tumor marker" may be run on request of a clinician who would specifically order the test (which may be part of a panel that includes all of the component/"predictor" tests), and thus the trigger would be a specific order. In contrast, a sepsis risk-screening algorithm intended to run in the background may be most useful as an alert for clinicians who may not be thinking about sepsis. In the case of the sepsis model, the trigger will need to be something more passive; for example, the model could be run every time a new relevant test result becomes available. Likewise, the algorithm output must be considered. For example, an abstract sepsis risk score may be of little value. A sepsis risk score would likely be more informative if accompanied by a narrative comment describing the degree of risk, the basis for the assessment, and a suggested clinical response (eg, orders for plasma lactate, blood cultures, antibiotics). Furthermore, a sepsis alert might be best communicated to a clinician as an interruptive alert in the patient's electronic chart; in contrast, the synthetic tumor marker could perhaps be displayed as a laboratory test result alongside other results.

Clinical informaticians may consider building alerts that directly allow for follow-up action; for example, an alert could include a single button click to order recommended follow-up studies. Finally, whereas some prediction models might be translated "as is" into the logic layer of a clinical algorithm, in other cases a trained prediction model might be used to provide clinical insights that are then used to guide the development of decision support logic more suitable for implementation.

A FEW ILLUSTRATIVE EXAMPLES

To provide a few examples of machine-learning knowledge discovery and translation to clinical algorithms, this section provides examples from the authors' own research. Baron and colleagues[25] used a type of supervised machine-learning known as recursive partitioning to automatically construct a decision tree to identify spuriously elevated plasma glucose results. They found that other analytes measured on the same tube of blood as the glucose can predict whether the glucose is spurious or real with a high degree of accuracy. However, in curating this knowledge into a clinical algorithm, the authors chose not to implement the decision trees as directly constructed. Rather, they used insights from the trees to generate a simplified flowchart optimized for usability and clinical safety and provided this to the technologists in their laboratory to use as a guide in spotting erroneous results. Likewise, Luo and colleagues[19] developed a framework to predict patient ferritin test results (a plasma biomarker of iron stores) using the results of laboratory tests performed alongside the ferritin on the same patient. They found that ferritin could usually be predicted with a high degree of accuracy, but that occasionally the model predicts a low ferritin suggestive of iron deficiency when the measured ferritin result is normal; in these cases, it seems that the algorithm's predictions may at least sometimes be more reflective of the patient's underlying iron status than the measured ferritin. Although the authors have not yet translated these findings into a clinical algorithm, they propose developing an algorithm that predicts ferritin in addition to measuring ferritin each time a ferritin test is ordered; when the predicted values are highly discrepant from the measured values, the measured values could be reported with a comment warning the clinician that the ferritin may not accurately represent the patient's iron status. As another example, Rosenbaum and Baron developed a machine-learning-based delta check algorithm that can look across changes in multiple test results to identify wrong blood in tube errors (ie, identify cases whereby the specimen was labeled with the wrong patient).[26]

IMPLEMENTATION OF ALGORITHMS

After developing a clinical algorithm, informaticians must implement the algorithm into practice for it to be of value in enhancing clinical care. In some cases it may be feasible to use clinical knowledge discovered through machine learning to develop an algorithm or insights intended for manual computation or application; clinical scoring algorithms, whereby various clinical criteria are worth various point values, or our aforementioned glucose example, are good examples of such manual algorithms. However, more complex algorithms and those intended for passive decision support must be implemented electronically. Although in certain limited cases it may be feasible to ask a clinician to input patient information into a "calculator" that computes the algorithm, in most cases, this will require too much time and effort for the algorithm to be much use; thus, implementation of most emerging decision support will require systems that can automatically extract predictor data from the EHR and communicate decision support back to clinicians through the EHR or closely integrated portals. Successful implementation in this context requires navigating technical, administrative, and educational challenges.

Technical Considerations

Two key technical challenges are (1) leveraging existing health information systems or developing and interfacing "bolt-on" portals for computation of clinical algorithms and (2) accessing, normalizing, and mapping EHR data for use as algorithm predictors. Regarding the first challenge of algorithm computation, solutions are available and in development, as discussed below. The second challenge related to data access and mapping is often solvable through manual work, as also discussed below; however, more general solutions are needed to make this process scalable and less resource-intensive.

Algorithm Computation

Historically, most traditional health information systems were not capable of directly implementing complex machine-learning algorithms. Although existing systems often offered various decision support functions, the logic of these was often limited to "if/then" criteria and/or simple arithmetical operations. Although it would be theoretically possible to implement simple algorithms such as basic decision trees or linear regression-based models using this more traditional CDS functionality, these systems would not be capable of computing more complex models. For example, the authors implemented a decision support alert designed to identify patient creatinine results that might be suggestive of acute kidney injury; although the desired underlying algorithm was quite straightforward, the authors had to develop complex workarounds to implement this within their hospital's laboratory information system.[8] Some vendors of health information systems are recognizing this shortcoming and are including modules capable of executing a compiled function of any computable form (assuming sufficient computing resources) within their core systems; however, these modules are at various stages of development and to the authors' knowledge, in many cases are not in wide use. Another solution is to build external decision support engines that interface with the EHR.[27–30]

The development of more robust interfacing standards may facilitate the practical implementation of external CDS engines. One standard that may be particularly valuable is the Fast Healthcare Interoperability Resources (FHIR) standard. Other references are available to provide a more comprehensive description of FHIR.[27,31,32] In brief, a basic building block of FHIR is a "Resource."[32] Resources are designed to provide a standard way to communicate various pieces of health information (eg, that a certain patient has a certain condition). Each resource contains a common set of metadata, in addition to a set of human-readable information.[32] The goal of FHIR is to build base resources that accommodate most common use cases. Remaining required content can be handled using a built-in extension mechanism.

One often overlooked consideration related to algorithm implementation is that, with most types of models, model training is much more computationally intensive than model application. Thus, a model can sometimes be trained offline using sophisticated computing resources and clusters, and can then be implemented within much less computationally powerful platforms.

Data Extraction and Mapping

Another challenge in the implementation of clinical algorithms is access and mapping data from the EHR into the predictor fields that are needed for the algorithm. For example, perhaps a patient's weight could exist in multiple fields within the EHR. For an algorithm to rely on patient weight, the various potential fields would need to be considered and mapped as possible inputs; the reliability of the information in each field would need to be considered and logic may be required to address conflicting information. Because these mapping issues will be system and case specific, details are outside the scope of this article, but, of course, the process can be complex. Likewise, extracting information from poorly structured health records can be particularly challenging; even when records are mapped to clinical standards (eg, LOINC, ICD, CPT, SNOMED), normalizing the various results for use in CDS can be complex and may require the use of various custom groupers or mapping tables, because there may be many codes that correspond to similar clinical features that could all be considered together for use in a model.

Testing, Validation, and Monitoring

A key step in algorithm implementation is testing and validation. Although the algorithm may have been extensively evaluated offline using retrospective data, the implementation itself includes many potential points of error and thus the implementation itself must be tested. Although the standards for clinical algorithm testing are poorly established, presumably most clinical algorithms (at a minimum) should be tested (as appropriate) using processes similar to those for more general health IT testing; details of health IT testing are outside the scope of this article. However, machine-learning-based clinical algorithms may present some unique testing challenges in so far as the algorithm underpinnings are often difficult to decipher, and it can thus be difficult to identify all of the edge cases that would ordinarily be tested.

Administrative and Educational Challenges

Many of the challenges to the effective implementation of artificially intelligent CDS are non-technical and involve primarily administrative or educational challenges. Administrative considerations include governance, regulation, medical-legal risk, funding, and financial impact. Implementing novel CDS into the EHR will usually require informaticians to obtain approvals from institutional health IT governance committees; as these emerging CDS technologies gain traction, institutional governance structures may need to adapt procedures to better evaluate and approve the implementation of these technologies. Likewise, regulatory and medical-legal issues may need to be addressed. The authors are certainly not lawyers or experts in these legal issues and thus are not qualified to include a detailed assessment in this article. However, in their experience, computational pathologists and those involved in computational pathology proposals and projects have expressed concerns regarding what regulatory requirements, such as US Food and Drug Administration approval, might be required for certain technologies intended for multi-institutional use and what the barriers to obtaining this might be. Likewise, informaticians have raised concerns regarding potential legal liability for adverse events for both the CDS developers and the clinician-users of the technology.

Widespread, successful implementation of emerging CDS technologies will require additional clinician education related to how best to interact with and apply recommendations from these systems; the authors envision the possibility that future medical school curricula will include teaching on how to evaluate CDS algorithms and their recommendations, similar to how evidence-based medicine curricula have historically taught physicians-in-training to evaluate clinical trials. To this end, informaticians may likewise need to develop clinical algorithms that are more transparent and easily understood by clinicians. Finally, like most technologies, health systems and the field as a whole will have to address the financial impacts and how to make these technologies financially sustainable.

SUMMARY

As discussed in this article, emerging approaches to CDS offer tremendous opportunity to enhance clinical practice and patient outcomes; however, numerous technical, administrative, and educational barriers remain. The authors expect that these barriers will be largely surmountable through clinical and engineering innovations and alterations to administrative processes and frameworks.

REFERENCES

1. Baron JM, Dighe AS. The role of informatics and decision support in utilization management. Clin Chim Acta 2014;427:196–201.
2. Kim JY, Dzik WH, Dighe AS, et al. Utilization management in a large urban academic medical center: a 10-year experience. Am J Clin Pathol 2011;135:108–18.
3. Baron JM, Dighe AS. Computerized provider order entry in the clinical laboratory. J Pathol Inform 2011;2:35.
4. Grisson R, Kim JY, Brodsky V, et al. A novel class of laboratory middleware. Promoting information flow and improving computerized provider order entry. Am J Clin Pathol 2010;133:860–9.
5. Henricks WH, Wilkerson ML, Castellani WJ, et al. Pathologists as stewards of laboratory information. Arch Pathol Lab Med 2015;139:332–7.
6. Sepulveda JL, Young DS. The ideal laboratory information system. Arch Pathol Lab Med 2013;137:1129–40.
7. Baron JM, Lewandrowski KB, Kamis IK, et al. A novel strategy for evaluating the effects of an electronic test ordering alert message: optimizing cardiac marker use. J Pathol Inform 2012;3:3.
8. Baron JM, Cheng XS, Bazari H, et al. Enhanced creatinine and estimated glomerular filtration rate reporting to facilitate detection of acute kidney injury. Am J Clin Pathol 2015;143:42–9.
9. Louis DN, Feldman M, Carter AB, et al. Computational pathology. Arch Pathol Lab Med 2016;41:41–50.
10. Louis DN, Gerber GK, Baron JM, et al. Computational pathology: an emerging definition. Arch Pathol Lab Med 2014;138:1133–8.
11. Shirts BH, Jackson BR, Baird GS, et al. Clinical laboratory analytics: challenges and promise for an emerging discipline. J Pathol Inform 2015;6:9.
12. Bastanlar Y, Ozuysal M. Introduction to machine learning. Methods Mol Biol 2014; 1107:105–28.
13. Hand DJ. Aspects of data ethics in a changing world: where are we now? Big Data 2018;6:176–90.
14. Mittelstadt BD, Floridi L. The ethics of big data: current and foreseeable issues in biomedical contexts. Sci Eng Ethics 2016;22:303–41.
15. Al-Hablani B. The use of automated SNOMED CT clinical coding in clinical decision support systems for preventive care. Perspect Health Inf Manag 2017;14:1f.
16. Ciolko E, Lu F, Joshi A. Intelligent clinical decision support systems based on SNOMED CT. Conf Proc IEEE Eng Med Biol Soc 2010;2010:6781–4.
17. Cornet R, de Keizer N. Forty years of SNOMED: a literature review. BMC Med Inform Decis Mak 2008;8(Suppl 1):S2.
18. Ahmadian L, van Engen-Verheul M, Bakhshi-Raiez F, et al. The role of standardized data and terminological systems in computerized clinical decision support systems: literature review and survey. Int J Med Inform 2011;80:81–93.
19. Luo Y, Szolovits P, Dighe AS, et al. Using machine learning to predict laboratory test results. Am J Clin Pathol 2016;145:778–88.

20. Luo Y, Szolovits P, Dighe AS, et al. 3D-MICE: integration of cross-sectional and longitudinal imputation for multi-analyte longitudinal clinical data. J Am Med Inform Assoc 2018;25:645–53.
21. Waljee AK, Mukherjee A, Singal AG, et al. Comparison of imputation methods for missing laboratory data in medicine. BMJ Open 2013;3 [pii:e002847].
22. Stekhoven DJ, Buhlmann P. MissForest–non-parametric missing value imputation for mixed-type data. Bioinformatics 2012;28:112–8.
23. van Buuren S, Boshuizen HC, Knook DL. Multiple imputation of missing blood pressure covariates in survival analysis. Stat Med 1999;18:681–94.
24. van Buuren S, Groothuis-Oudshoorn K. Mice: multivariate imputation by chained equations in R. J Stat Softw 2011;45:1–67.
25. Baron JM, Mermel CH, Lewandrowski KB, et al. Detection of preanalytic laboratory testing errors using a statistically guided protocol. Am J Clin Pathol 2012; 138:406–13.
26. Rosenbaum MW, Baron JM. Using machine learning-based multianalyte delta checks to detect wrong blood in tube errors. Am J Clin Pathol 2018;150:555–66.
27. Mandel JC, Kreda DA, Mandl KD, et al. SMART on FHIR: a standards-based, interoperable apps platform for electronic health records. J Am Med Inform Assoc 2016;23:899–908.
28. Aronson S, Mahanta L, Ros LL, et al. Information technology support for clinical genetic testing within an Academic Medical center. J Pers Med 2016;6 [pii:E4].
29. Aronson SJ, Rehm HL. Building the foundation for genomics in precision medicine. Nature 2015;526:336–42.
30. Mandl KD, Mandel JC, Kohane IS. Driving innovation in health systems through an apps-based information economy. Cell Syst 2015;1:8–13.
31. Boussadi A, Zapletal E. A fast healthcare interoperability resources (FHIR) layer implemented over i2b2. BMC Med Inform Decis Mak 2017;17:120.
32. Health Level Seven International. FHIR. Available at: http://hl7.org/fhir. Accessed November 12, 2018.

Moving?

Make sure your subscription moves with you!

To notify us of your new address, find your **Clinics Account Number** (located on your mailing label above your name), and contact customer service at:

Email: journalscustomerservice-usa@elsevier.com

800-654-2452 (subscribers in the U.S. & Canada)
314-447-8871 (subscribers outside of the U.S. & Canada)

Fax number: 314-447-8029

Elsevier Health Sciences Division
Subscription Customer Service
3251 Riverport Lane
Maryland Heights, MO 63043

*To ensure uninterrupted delivery of your subscription, please notify us at least 4 weeks in advance of move.

Printed and bound by CPI Group (UK) Ltd, Croydon, CR0 4YY

03/10/2024

01040483-0012